Acupuncture Styles in Current Practice

Martin Wang, MD. , PhD

Millwoods Acupuncture Center, Edmonton, Canada

Email: Wenqiw57@hotmail.com

Abstract: There are many different styles of acupuncture in current practice. Some follow the traditional acupuncture meridian system, some do not. Each style has its advantages and disadvantages in clinical application. As an acupuncturist, it is better to know the difference among the various acupuncture styles, so as to choose the proper style of acupuncture for the treatment. For acupuncture researchers, it is necessary to know that the textbook style of acupuncture, which is currently under extensive study for its clinic efficacy, is only one of several acupuncture styles, though it is used more than other styles in clinics. For research into the efficacy of a given acupuncture style, it is necessary to follow the exact procedure that is requested for that style of acupuncture, from the diagnosis to the treatment. For research on the acupuncture mechanism, it should be kept in mind that any hypothesis for the mechanism needs to explain the whole acupuncture style, not only parts of it.

Key words: Acupuncture, technique, style, meridian, Holographic theory

Contents

Introduction 6

I.   Classification of acupuncture styles 7

1. Meridian-based whole body acupuncture group 7

(1)   Textbook acupuncture style (教材针灸法) 7

(2)   Time-circle acupuncture style (子午流注针法) 9

(3)   Wang Wen-Yuan Balancing acupuncture (王文远平衡针法) 12

(4)   Tan Wu-Bian Balancing acupuncture (谭无边平衡针法) 12

(5)   Li Bai-Song Eight-words acupuncture (李柏松八字疗法) 13

(6)   Chen Zhao Crane-pine Yi Xue[0] acupuncture (陈照鹤松易学针法) 16

(7)   Liu Ji-ling new one-needle acupuncture (刘吉领新一针疗法) 17

(8)   Zhang Xian-Chen Hand-Foot Three-needle acupuncture style (张显臣手足三针疗法) 18

(9)   Jin Rui Three-needle acupuncture style (靳三针疗法) 19

(10)   Fu Zhong-Hua Floating acupuncture style (符中华浮针疗法) 20

(11)   Zhao Wu-Rong Flying acupuncture style (赵武荣飞针针法) 22

(12)   Li Jin-Niu Five-element acupuncture style (李金牛五行生克针灸) 23

(13)   Ma Xiao-Ping Five-element acupuncture style (马小平补北泻南法) 25

(14)   Yangming Wuxing acupuncture (阳明五行针法) 25

(15)   Mang acupuncture style (蟒针,芒针) 25

(16)   Guo Zhi-Chen Eight-point acupuncture style (郭志辰八穴针法) 26

(17)   Pan Xiao-Chuan Classical acupuncture style (潘晓川古典针灸) 28

(18)   Korea Sha-Am Five-element acupuncture (韩国舍岩五行针法) 30

(19)   Korea Li Ji-Ma Four-diagram acupuncture style (李济马太极四象针灸) ..30

(20)   Nora Five-element acupuncture style (Nora 五行针法) 31

(21)   Japanese acupuncture 39

(22)   Various special manipulating techniques of acupuncture 40

2. Acupuncture styles only partly following traditional meridian 41

(1)   Dong Jing-Chang extraordinary point acupuncture style (董氏奇穴疗法)41

(2)   Ke Shang-Zhi Distance-meridian acupressure therapy (柯尚志远络疗法)44

(3)   Han Wen-Zhi One-needle Acupuncture style (韩文治一针疗法) 48

(4)   Zhang Xin-Shu wrist-ankle acupuncture style (腕踝针法) 48

(5)   Western style of Medicine Acupuncture 50

3.   Local acupuncture style (局部针法) 51

(1)   Auricular acupuncture style (耳针) 51

(2)   Scalp acupuncture (头皮针) 52

(2.1) Jiao Sun-Fa Scalp acupuncture style （焦顺发头皮针) 53

(2.2) Fang Yun-Peng scalp acupuncture style (方云鹏头皮针) 53

(2.3) Zhu Ming-Qing scalp acupuncture style (朱明清头皮针) 54

(2.4) Liu Bing-Quan scalp acupuncture style (刘炳权八卦头针) 56

(2.5) Tang Song-Yan scalp acupuncture style (汤颂延头针) 57

(2.6) Lin Xue-Jian scalp acupuncture style (林学俭头针刺激新区) 57

(2.7) Yu Chang-De scalp acupuncture style (俞昌德头针) 58

(2.8) Jin Rui scalp acupuncture style (靳瑞头针) 58

(2.9) Toshikatsu scalp acupuncture style (山元敏胜新头针) 58

(3)   Face acupuncture style (面针) 59

(3.1) Traditional facial acupuncture (传统面针) 59

(3.2) New facial acupuncture (新面针) 60

(4)   Peng Jin-Shan Eye acupuncture style (彭静山眼针疗法) 62

(5)   Nose acupuncture style (鼻针) 63

(6)   Tongue acupuncture style (舌针) 64

(7)   Mouth acupuncture style (口针) 65

(8)   Ren-zhong acupuncture style (人中针) 65

(9)   Foot acupuncture style (足针) 66

(10)   Fang Ben-Zheng Foot region acupuncture style (足象针) 67

(11)   Hand acupuncture (手针针法) 68

(12)   Hand region acupuncture style (手象针针法) 68

(13)   Yu Hao Yin-Yang Nine-acupuncture style (余浩阴阳九针) 69

(14)   Ma Chun-Hui Small Six-He acupuncture (马春晖小六合针法) 71

(15)   Ge Qin-Fu Taiji Si-He acupuncture style (葛钦甫腹部太极六合针法) 73

(16)   Dr. Bo Zhi-Yun Abdominal acupuncture style (薄智云腹针疗法) 74

(17)   Sun Shen-Tian Abdominal Acupuncture style (孙申田腹针疗法) 76

(18)   Qi Yong Navel acupuncture (齐永脐针) 78

(19)   Holographic acupuncture system (全息针灸体系) 83

(20)   Feng Ning-Han Nine-place Acupuncture style (冯宁汉九宫针法) 85

(21)   Guan Zhen-Zai Nine-Palace Acupuncture style (管正斋九宫针法) 86

(22)   Along-spine acupuncture style (脊针针法) 87

3.   Local acupuncture styles for local diseases 88

(1)   A Shi point acupuncture (阿是穴疗法) 88

(2)   Release point acupuncture (反阿是穴疗法) 89

(3)   Trigger point (扳机点疗法) 89

(4)   Liu Nong-Yu Sinew acupuncture (刘农虞筋针疗法) 90

II.   Characteristics of current acupuncture styles 90

1.   Acupuncture points to be stimulated 91

2.   Diagnosis directing the selection of the acupuncture point 93

3.   Steady point versus dynamic points 93

4.   Accuracy of acupuncture points 93

5.   Depth of needle insertion 94

6.   Intensity of treatment stimulation 94

7.   Healing efficiency of acupuncture styles 95

8.   Whole body acupuncture versus local acupuncture 96

III.   Acupuncture research 96

Conclusion 99

Our Publications 101

Introduction

There are many styles of acupuncture in ancient and current practice. The acupuncture manipulation described in older acupuncture textbooks is usually limited to several common styles of acupuncture. However, there are many styles of acupuncture in practice, especially in China. It would be helpful for both acupuncturists and acupuncture researchers in Western countries to know this important fact in order to gain better acupuncture efficacy and research products.

In this chapter, I summarized a variety of acupuncture manipulation methods in practice for acupuncturists' reference and for researchers who have little or no clinical experience and who have limited theoretical knowledge of acupuncture. Hopefully, the contents of this chapter help achieve better clinical and research outcomes.

I will mainly focus on the needle-based acupuncture styles. I will not focus on some modified acupuncture or acupuncture-like therapies such as point injection, fire acupuncture, electro-acupuncture, bundle needle, dermal needle, bleeding needle, small knife-needle technique and so on. I also exclude information on other techniques that are commonly used in Traditional Chinese Medicine (TCM) and acupuncture clinics, e.g., various moxibustion, cupping, Hans machine, TENS, acupressure, tapping, TDP, or bleeding therapy. Because of space limitation, I will only make a brief introduction to each style of acupuncture here and it is impossible to explain the concepts (such as Five-element theory, Five-shu theory, Time-circle theory, Nine-palace theory, Eight-diagram theory, the relationship between the meridians in the body, and so on) and terminology used in each acupuncture style.

For those who are interested in any of the specific styles of acupuncture, I recommend reading the relevant books or journal articles in detail, or obtaining special training. The names of acupuncture points used in this book are indicated with Chinese Pinyin, not the letter-number as used in an acupuncture textbook, since many acupuncture points cannot be easily indicated by this letter-number system.

In the below contents, I regards all of the founders of the acupuncture styles as "Doctor" (Dr.) although many of them may not have graduated from any medical school with a medical degree.

I. Classification of acupuncture styles

1. Meridian-based whole body acupuncture group
According to the principle of acupuncture points, the acupuncture style can be separated into whole body acupuncture groups and local acupuncture groups.

(1) Textbook acupuncture style (教材针灸法)

This is the acupuncture style that students in acupuncture schools in Western countries or China learn from their textbook.[1, 2] We do not use "traditional Chinese acupuncture" to name this style of acupuncture because there are many other types of acupuncture that should also belong to the "traditional" acupuncture group, but they are not introduced in the textbook.

Many of the contents that have been introduced in the textbook, such as Time-circle acupuncture theory and Five-shu acupuncture, are not suggested in the treatment plan for the treatment of a disease (see below) in the textbook. Most of the acupuncturists who graduate from acupuncture schools are neither using such Time-circle acupuncture technique nor the Five-element theory in the Five-shu style.

Therefore we define the acupuncture style that uses mostly the textbook-suggested treatment plan, as textbook acupuncture.[1] In the textbook acupuncture, the acupuncture points are selected mostly from traditional meridians.[3]

In the textbook acupuncture style, acupuncturist uses either meridian diagnosis or TCM organ diagnosis (to tell if a disease is in the Yin and Yang aspect, if it is on the body's surface or inside the body, if it belongs to Cold or Hotness, or if it has sufficient or insufficient status) to guide the selection of the acupuncture points.

---

[1] This is not to look down the acupuncture system introduced in the text book, but anyway, it is only a part of the whole "traditional Chinese acupuncture". This is similar to the Chinese herbal therapy: in the text book of Chinese herbology, the Shang Han Lun is also introduced, but in the suggested treatment plan for almost all the diseases, the way of herbal therapy in the Shang Han Lun is not recommended, so that we still separate the herbal therapy of the Shang Han Lun from the textbook herbology.

For example, for the treatment of lower back pain, when using the meridian diagnosis, if the disease is in the Urine bladder meridian, acupuncture points are mostly chosen from the Urine bladder meridian as basic points: Shen Shu, Weizhong. With further organ diagnosis from TCM, if the lower back pain is due to Cold-Wetness, we use the Yaoyangguan point. If it is due to denegation we use Geshu and Ciliao. If it is due to Kidney deficiency, we use Mingmen, Zhishi and Taixi. To enhance the healing effect, it is also recommended to use some special points such as Jijia, and the A Shi point (painful spot).

For the treatment of headaches or migraines, the choice of acupuncture points depends on the location of the headache (the meridian diagnosis), or TCM organ diagnosis, or a combination of both.

For a headache on the top of the head, use point Baihui, Tongtian, Xingjian; on the front of the head, use point Shangxing, Touwei, Hegu; on the side of the head, use point Shuaigu, Taiyang, Xiaxi; on the rear of head, use Houding, Tianzhu, Kunlun. If the headache is diagnosed from TCM point of view as Liver-Yang overwhelming, use point Fengchi, Baihui, Xuanlu, Xiaxi and Xingjian; if it is Qi and Blood deficiency, use Baihui, Qihai, Ganshu, Pishu, Shenshu, Hegu, and Zusanli; if it is Blood stagnation, use Shangxing, Touwei, Shuaigu, Taiyang, Houding. To enhance healing, the A Shi point can be used too.

For the treatment of asthma, it belongs to the disorder in the Lung system, so the Hand Lung meridian is chosen. Again, if it is diagnosed according to TCM as Phlegm-heat, other acupuncture points are also used too: point Feishu (on the Du meridian), Dingchuan (Extra point), Tiantu (Ren meridian), Chize (Lung meridian), Fenglong (Foot Yangming meridian).[4]

For the same kind of diagnosis as Phlegm-heat type of asthma, the suggested acupuncture points may different from textbook to textbook. For example, also for the treatment of Phlegm-heart type of asthma introduced by another acupuncture textbook,[5] the points suggested are Chize (Lung meridian), Zhongfu (Lung meridian), Quchi (Large intestine meridian), Fenglong (Stomach meridian), Dazhui (Du meridian).

In fact, there are several types of asthma with the TCM diagnosis, including Wind-cold, Phlegm-heat, Lung-deficiency, and Kidney-deficiency. Therefore, for a group of patients with asthma, their diagnosis from the TCM point of view could be very different, so that the acupuncture treatment should also be different in terms of the choice of acupuncture points and how to manipulate the needles, etc. To use the same way of acupuncture for the treatment of all the patients with the same Western medicine-diagnosed diseases (such as knee arthritis or sciatic pain), is the way of Western style of acupuncture, and is not typical TCM acupuncture.

Depending on whether the disease belongs to overwhelming (e.g. excessive) or weak (deficiency) of Qi in the meridian(s), the needles have to be manipulated as nourishing or depleting in technique.

The acupuncture points used can also be on points that do not belong to any meridian. These are called extra-ordinary points. In recent years, more and more such extra-ordinary points have been found[6, 7] and the total number of extra points might be more than traditional points in the meridians.

Sometimes, especially if pain is mostly in the muscle-tenden system, we also use needles around the painful spot or on the spot. This technique has been developed into a trigger point treatment as well.

Whether to use only the traditional acupuncture points, the extra-ordinary points, the spot points, or a combination of them, depends on the type of disease, and the experience and habit of the acupuncturists.

(2) Time-circle acupuncture style (子午流注针法)

This style of acupuncture also uses the acupuncture points in the traditional meridians, but the way of choosing the acupuncture point is different.[8]

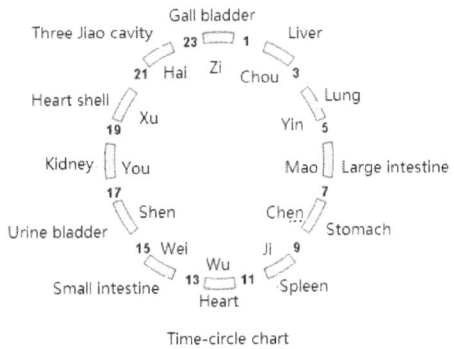

Time-circle chart

The fingers in chart is time of the day

Figure 1. Time circle of life energy flow in body during a day.[9]

9

It is believed in TCM that the life energy in the body is in dynamic flowing as a circle. At a given point in time, the life energy flow is stronger in one meridian and weaker in another meridian. The intensity of the life energy in the meridians is related to the year, the day and the hour of the day. For example, the life energy is overwhelming in the Lung meridian between 3 am and 5 am and, at the same time, it is weak in the Urine bladder meridian (Figure 1). The acupuncture points are chosen based on the time of the month, the day, or the hours of the day.

There are more than 10 ways to apply this time-circle theory in acupuncture practice. To use it, firstly we need a meridian diagnosis to identify the disease and meridian it belongs to. Secondly, we need the knowledge of the Chinese expression of the year, the month, the day and the hour of the day, Five-element theory, Five-shu points, and more.

The easiest and most popularly used method is the Na Zi (time of day) method. For example, chronic cough is diagnosed as a disorder in the Lung meridian. The energy in the Lung meridian is overwhelming between 3 am and 5 am, so we can stimulate acupuncture in the Lung meridian every day between the 3 am and the 5 am. Similarly, for the treatment of insomnia (poor sleep), if it is diagnosed as a disconnection between the Heart and the Kidney, the acupuncturist can stimulate any acupuncture points in the Heart meridian between 11 am and 1 pm, and in the Kidney meridian between 5 pm and 7 pm.

More specifically for the chronic cough, if it is diagnosed as Lung Qi deficiency, the acupuncturist can follow the Five-element theory with the Five-shu acupuncture on the given meridian (Figure 2). This acupuncture also is performed every day between the 3 am and 5 am. For the Lung Qi deficiency, the acupuncturist can stimulate the Soil point in the Lung meridian (every meridian has five points, which belong to one of the five elements: Wood, Fire, Soil, Metal and Water), which is the Taiyuan point (with nourishing technique of needle manipulation). However, if the cough is diagnosed as Lung excess, the acupuncturist stimulates the Water point on the Lung meridian with depleting technique, which is the Chize point. To nourish the Lung (Metal) meridian, the acupuncturist can also chose to stimulate the Soil point in the Soil meridian (Spleen meridian), which is the Taibei (Soil point). To deplete the Lung meridian (Metal), the acupuncturist can also deplete the

Water point in the Water meridian (Kidney meridian), which is the Yingu point (Water point).

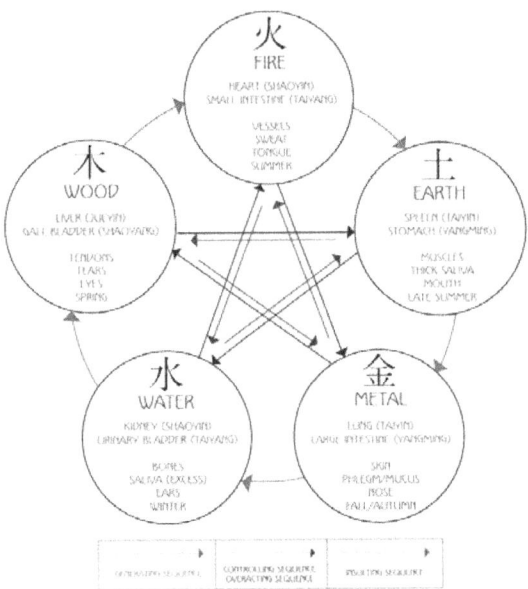

Figure 2. Relationship between five elements in traditional Five-element theory.[10]

If it is difficult for patients to have acupuncture during the optimal time period, or if it is hard to diagnose the excess or deficiency of the disease, or if the disease is acute, the acupuncturist can just stimulate the Self point or the Primary point of the meridian.[(2)] For example in the same cough treatment, the acupuncturist can stimulate the Self point (Metal) or the Primary point (Metal) of the Lung meridian, both of which, in the Lung meridian, are the Taiyuan point (Metal).

This way of choosing acupuncture points is not used popularly among acupuncturists either in China or in the Western world, though it is traditionally introduced in the textbook of acupuncture. However, there are experts in the use of this Time-circle acupuncture.[11 , 12 , 13 , 14] Though there is doubt from some acupuncturists about its certainty and usefulness in acupuncture practice,[15,16, 17] several acupuncture clinical studies suggested that when using either the Time-circle acupuncture along with textbook acupuncture,[18, 19] or when using the Time-circle acupuncture alone,[20, 21, 22, 23] compared with using textbook acupunc-

---

[(2)] Every meridian has its Self point and Primary point.

ture alone, the Time-circle acupuncture worked better than the text-book acupuncture.

(3) Wang Wen-Yuan Balancing acupuncture (王文远平衡针法)

This style of acupuncture[24] can be called Dr. Wang Wen-Yuan Balancing acupuncture style because it was developed by Dr. Wang Wen-Yuan. The acupuncture points are also selected from the whole of the body following Mirror theory, most of the time. It is said that 80% of diseases can be treated with only one acupuncture point. Totally it needs only 38 acupuncture points. The locations of the points do not need to be exactly correct, but needles should be on the correct distributing line of the correlated nerve.

The Dr. Wang Wen-Yuan style utilizes the acupuncture Deqi sensation by pulling-inserting technique, so there is no need for nourishing-depleting technique. The needle is taken out once it is felt by the patient. Retention of the needle is not required.

With this style of acupuncture, insertion is fast, and take-out is also fast. Whole treatment is within 3 seconds.

(4) Tan Wu-Bian Balancing acupuncture (谭无边平衡针法)

This style of acupuncture was developed by Dr. Tan Wu-Bian.[25, 26] It uses meridian diagnosis (not traditional organ diagnosis of TCM). Acupuncture points are chosen from the same meridian or other meridians, on the same side of the body or the other side of the body, but do not use the diseased spot.

For example, if the pain is on the lower part of the right front arm, the acupuncturist diagnoses that the pain is on the right Hand Yangming meridian. Therefore, the acupuncturist could choose a positively active point on the Left Foot Yangming meridian (e.g. the same name but on Foot and on opposite), or choose a positively active point on the Left Foot Jueyin meridian (e.g. the By-pass meridian),[(3)] or choose the positive point on the Taiyin meridian on the left arm (e.g. the Surface-inside relationship between the sick meridian and the treated meridian).

The location of the point on these chosen meridians follows the mirror theory. It is to stimulate the active point, not the traditional acupunc-

---

[(3)] The Yangming and Jueyin, the Shaoyin and Shaoyang, the Taiyin and Taiyang, are bypass meridian relationships.

ture points on the meridians. The active points are the points at which the patient feels pain when pressed by acupuncturists. This style of acupuncture also uses Time-circle theory to choose active points for the treatment.

After each treatment, the painful active spot might disappear (the original pain usually becomes much less), but may have a new painful spot later. It is necessary to re-evaluate the meridian and stimulate the active spot. Repeat each time until the original pain completely subsides. This rule is similarly used with Jing Fang (e.g. the herbal formula introduced in book *Shang Han Lun*) where the symptoms are removed one by one as layer after layer.

(5) Li Bai-Song Eight-words acupuncture (李柏松八字疗法)

This style of acupuncture was developed by acupuncturist Li Bai-Son (1938-2010). The eight Chinese words are 阴阳、相对、平衡、反应. The words mean Yin and Yang, relativity, balance, and reaction. These are the characteristics of this style of acupuncture.[27]

This style of acupuncture separates the body into several units: head, neck, trunk and limbs (both arms and both legs are each one unit). First, the acupuncturist needs to determine the painful (or sick) part of the body. Second, it is necessary to find reflecting zone (or reflecting spot(s)) of the painful spot in the same unit (Figure 3, 4).

For example, if the pain is on the lower back, it is necessary to find the reflecting area on the body trunk. If the pain is on arm, it is necessary to find the reflecting zone in the limb unit. If there is headache, it is necessary to find the reflecting zone in the head (not on the truck or limb unit).

The principle in finding the reflecting zone is that "the reflecting zone is crossly opposite on other side of the unit". To find the reflecting zones for head, neck and body trunk, follow the "reverse mirror" theory, and for limbs, follow the "mirror theory".

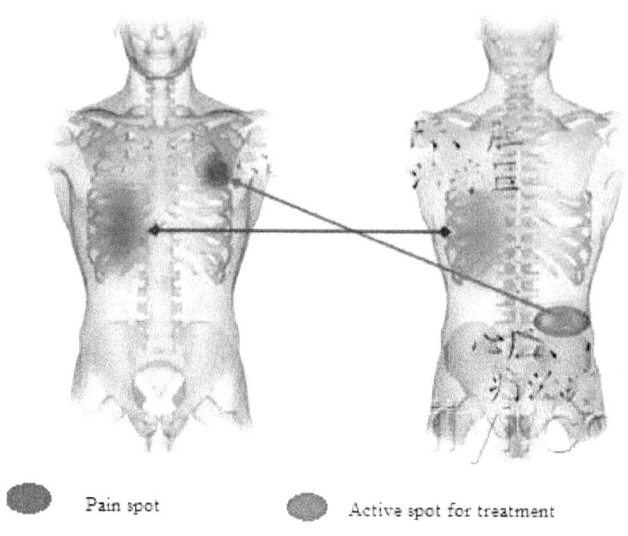

Pain spot   Active spot for treatment

Figure 3. Treatment of pain in the heart and liver area in the Li Bai-Song Eight-word balancing therapy. [28]

For example, if the pain is on the right and inner side of the front of the arm, the reflecting zone would be on back side of calf of left leg.[(4)] If the pain is on the lower back, its reflecting zone would be on the upper part of sternum. The exception is that the reflecting zone for the top of the head is on the perineal region. For the treatment of cervical spondylopathy, the reflecting zone could be on or around the synchondroses pubis. The reflecting zone for prostatitis, dysmenorrhea, and uterus fibroid, is on or around the spinous process of the seventh cervical vertebrae.

Again, it is necessary to find a sensitive spot(s) in the reflecting zone. This can be done by rubbing the zone with alcohol on cotton, in order to find a red color spot. This sensitive spot may or may not be located on traditional meridians. Generally speaking, the sensitive points will only work for diseases in the same unit. This means that acupuncturist does not try to find a reflecting zone on the arms or legs to solve diseases on the head or body trunk. Note, the active spot in this style of acupuncture is the color spot after rubbing, not the painful spot upon

---

[(4)] For the yin and yang zones in the body, refer
to :http://blog.sina.com.cn/s/blog_6383a68a0102e3sg.html

pressing by acupuncturist (e.g. not the pain spot as in the Tan Wu-Bian Balancing acupuncture above).

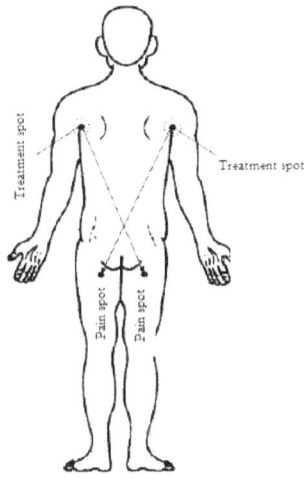

Figure 4. Treatment of pain in the rear of hip area in the Li Bai-Song Eight-words balancing therapy. [28]

Along with treatment and improvement of the disease, the sensitive spot may change its location and numbers. Therefore, it is said that any part of the body may be an acupuncture point and that acupuncture points are dynamic points.

After locating sensitive spots, use acupuncture to stimulate them.[5] Basically, it is necessary to stimulate so deep as to touch the bone membrane (except to treat shallow skin diseases, in which the stimulation is shallow too). It is painful stimulation.

To enhance the healing effect, it is necessary to also stimulate some "high energy" acupuncture points, such as Dazhui, Baihui, Qugu, Shenshu, Changqiang, the Common-Cold-three-needle points, and several points around the inner side and outer side of ankle.

It has been admitted that treatment as such could reduce the pain within a very short time, but also that the pain may come back again (re-

---

[5] The points can also be stimulated by moxibustion, finger press, Guasha, herbal patch, etc.

bound). To solve this problem, it has been suggested that the acupuncturist also includes a traditional Chinese medicine diagnosis and performs acupuncture on the related reflecting zone. For example, if a pain on the leg is diagnosed by TCM as a Liver problem, the acupuncturist will also stimulate the acupuncture points on the liver reflecting zone.[6]

(6) Chen Zhao Crane-pine Yi Xue[7] acupuncture (陈照鹤松易学针法)

This acupuncture style was created by Dr. Chen Zhao[29, 30] There are several ways to choose acupuncture points for treatment:

(1). Surface-inner related meridian (八卦成列). For example, if the pain is on the Yuji point (thenar muscles) on the left hand, which belongs to the Hand Taiyin meridian, the acupuncturist chooses the Hegu point on the right hand. Hequ belongs to Hand Yangming meridian, which has a surface-inner relationship with the Hand Taiyin meridian.

(2). Same-name meridian of the surface-inner related meridian (刚柔相摩). For example in the same case with pain in the Yuji point on the left hand, which belong to Hand Taiyin meridian, the acupuncturist can choose acupuncture points on the Foot Yangming meridian. Hand Yangming has a surface-inner relationship with the Taiyin meridian, so the acupuncturist chooses Foot Yangming meridian, rather than the Hand Yangming meridian.

(3). Same-name meridian (八卦相荡). In the same example above, the sick meridian is the Hand Yangming, so the acupuncturist then chooses the Foot Yangming meridian. The two meridians are the same name: Yangming.

(4). Four-diagram acupuncture (四局针法). The three meridians in the inner side of the arm are called Fire diagram; the three meridians in the outside of the arm are called Wood diagram; the three meridians in the inner side of the leg are called Metal diagram; and the three meridians in the back and outside of leg are called Water diagram.

---

[6] The liver zone however is designed according to the anatomic organ location, not TCM concept of liver.

[7] Yi Xue also means Yi Jing. It is a knowledge system for prediction of changes.

The principle for the choice of meridian for the treatment is this: if the sick meridian is in the Fire diagram, use acupuncture points on the Metal diagram; if the sick meridian belongs to the Metal diagram, choose acupuncture points in the Fire diagram.

Similarly, if the sick meridian is in the Wood diagram, the acupuncturist chooses acupuncture points in the Water diagram and if the sick meridian is in the Water diagram, chooses acupuncture points in the Wood diagram. All in all, it means that if the sick meridian belongs to the Yin meridian in the arm, the acupuncturist chooses acupuncture points also in the Yin meridian but on the leg. If the sick meridian is on the Yang meridian on the arm, the acupuncturist chooses acupuncture points also in the Yang meridian, but on the leg. Just pay attention that if the sick meridian is on the hand, the acupuncturist chooses to treat the meridian on the leg, and, if the sick meridian is on the left, the acupuncturist choose to treat the meridian on the right side.[8]

(5). Eight-diagram theory. It has been summarized by other acupuncturists[29] that this acupuncture style has principles in the selection of acupuncture points which mostly follow Eight-diagram theory.[9]

(7) Liu Ji-ling new one-needle acupuncture (刘吉领新一针疗法)

This style[31] is similar to Wang Wen-Yuan One-needle style. The acupuncture points are chosen from the opposite meridian. The acupuncture points are mostly located on traditional meridians. It does not require Deqi sensation. The needle sensation is very mild.

This style is suitable for the treatment of various symptoms such as headaches, spondylosis, neck-shoulder syndrome, tennis elbow, numbness in hands or feet, lumber spondylosis, lumber strain, pyriformis syndrome, various knee arthritis, ankle pain, and various bruise or strains.[32]

---

[8] It can also be understood as: the three Yang meridians treat disease in three Yang meridians in opposite (arm versus leg, left side versus right side).
[9] It was summarized to have more than 13 ways of choosing acupuncture points.

(8) Zhang Xian-Chen Hand-Foot Three-needle acupuncture style (张显臣手足三针疗法)

This style of acupuncture only uses three needles, either on the hands or feet each time (and rarely uses six needles on both hands and feet).[33] The tree acupuncture points on the hand are: Jiangu, Zhongzhu, Houxi. The three points on the foot are: Taichong, Neiting, and Zulinqi (Figure 5). It would be better to find and use sensitive or tender spot(s) around these acupuncture points. The needle tip for Zhongzhu is towards the finger. Those for Taichong, Neitin and Zulinqi are towards the ankle. The hand's three needles are used to treat disease over the hip. The foot's three needles are for disease below the hip level. Select the acupuncture points on the sick side of the body. If the pain is in middle of the body, select left side points for male and right side points for female. If the pain is in the middle (such as on the spine line), use acupuncture points on both sides.

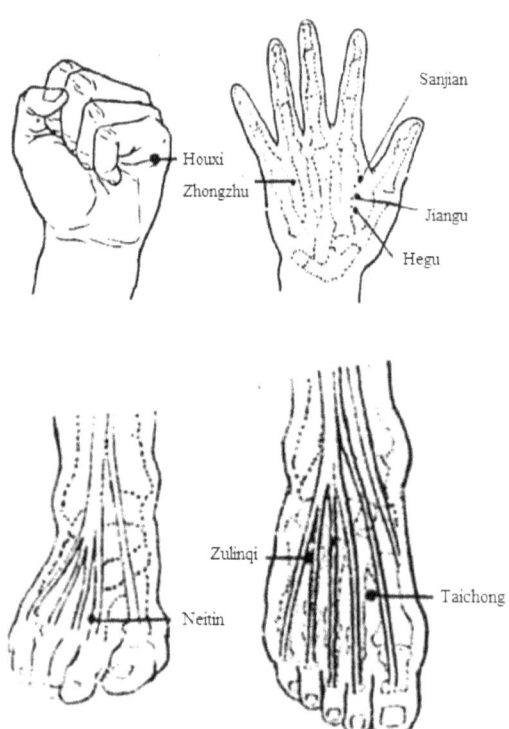

Figure 5. Hand three needles and Fee three needles in Zhang Xian-Chen three needle acupuncture.[34]

Find the most sour-pain spot on or around these points (press the skin with a hard material, such as a probe) on the sick side of the body. Stimulate the sensitive spot with acupuncture needles.

It is necessary that the needle is inserted very fast. Twist (three times in either direction) and pull once very quickly. Repeat this depletion technique twice to get Deqi sensation. Then pull up on the needle until it is nearly out of the skin (but not out of the skin). Change the direction of the needle tip to another direction that is parallel to the meridian, so as to stimulate the neighbor acupuncture points on the same meridian. Repeat the depletion technique twice for the acupuncture point on each direction. The patient could feel a lot of pain during the treatment. Most of the needles are inserted at oblique angles (15 to 30 degree to skin), except for Jiangu and Houxi, which should be inserted vertically.

Deqi sensation occurs very fast. Once the Deqi sensation occurs from the last point, the needle is taken out. The whole treatment lasts for only one to two minutes. For this acupuncture style, the Deqi sensation is very strong. After taking out the needle, ask the patient to move the sick part of the body. The three acupuncture points are used one by one. If the pain is gone completely with the first needle, do not continue with the second acupuncture point.

(9) Jin Rui Three-needle acupuncture style (靳三针疗法)

This Three-needle acupuncture was developed by Dr. Jin Rui.[35] It uses three needles as a group in each small part of the body for the treatment (Figure 6). For example, there are feet three-needle, hand three-needle, eye three-needles, brain three-needle, intelligence three-needle, and so on.

In the treatment, the different three-needle groups may be combined. For example, for the treatment of arthritis in both hands, the three-needle in the left hand is used with another three-needle in the right hand. For the treatment of dizziness, the sedation three-needle is combined with the dizziness-pain three-needle. For the treatment of paralysis, the shoulder three-needle, hand three-needle, and the brain three-needle might be used the same time.

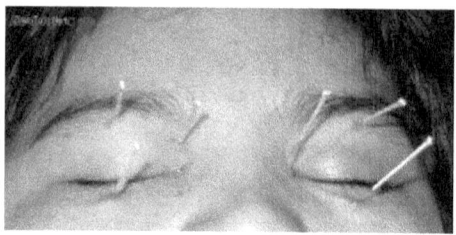

Figure 6. Eye three-needles in the Jin Three-needle group.[35]

The acupuncture points belong to the traditional meridians. The Deqi sensation is required.

(10)   Fu Zhong-Hua Floating acupuncture style (符中华浮针疗法)

This style of acupuncture was developed by Dr. Fu Zhong-Hua in year 1996.[36] It is also called Fu's Subcutaneous Needling (FSN).[10]

The selection of the acupuncture point also follows the meridian system. However, after being inserted into the skin, the body of the needle should be only between the skin and the fiber membrane that folds the muscle, and does not at all penetrate into the muscle (Figure 7). In other words, the needle is within the loose connective tissue.

The needle, which is thicker than and ordinary acupuncture needle, is mostly applied around the painful spot (the tip of the needle points towards the pain spot). The needle is manipulated but does not aim to let the patient feel anything (e.g. no typical Deqi acupuncture sensation is desired). The needle is retained in the loose connective tissue for a longer time,[11] usually 6-24 hours.[37] With the needle in the loose connective tissue, the patient is asked to move the affected body part to increase the healing effect. Each treatment needs only one to two needles. For chronic pain, we need only 3 to 4 times of treatment.

---

[10] This type of acupuncture system has been translated as Floating Acupuncture、Fu's Acupuncture，Fu Needling、Floating Needling, and now, mostly as Fu's Subcutaneous Needling.

[11] The pain can subside very quickly. However if the needle is released after that, the pain may come back again (rebound pain), so that retention of needle (or plastic tube) in the subcutaneous layer is required.

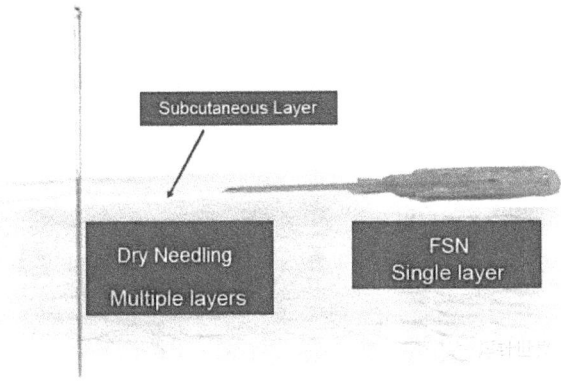

Figure 7. Working layer of Fu Zhong-Hua subcutaneous needle acu-puncture.[38]

Generally speaking, the diseases that can be treated by FSN are similar to most of traditional acupuncture, such as chronic headache, cervical spondylosis, periarthritis of the shoulder, tennis elbow, peritendinitis, carpal tunnel syndrome, prolapse of lumbar intervertebral disc, lumbar muscle degeneration, gonarthritis, old injury of the ankle joint, femoral head necrosis, ankylosing spondylitis, cholecystitis and gallstone, chronic stomach pain, urinary stone, chronic accessory inflammation, cervicitis, dysmenorrhea, intractable facial paralysis, and so on.

The hypothesis for the FSN is that the loose connective tissue in be-tween the skin and muscle is the main channel for the transportation and movement of material, energy and signal-information in the body. Any block to the channel would affect the transportation of these life element movements in the loose connective tissue. The block would decrease the threshold of the nerve to cause painful feelings. Removing the block with a TSN needle would re-open the channel, and restore the pain threshold and stop the pain. This is pretty much the same mechanism used to explain the function of various local therapies, such as trigger point therapy, anti-trigger point therapy, small needle-knife, as well as the Wrist-ankle acupuncture therapy.

Because the needle is different from traditional acupuncture needle and the needle is moved in the loose connective tissue in a swipe manner, rather than the vertical insertion of the needles typical in traditional acupuncture, the FSN therapy can be regarded as a mild surgical operation, similar to the small needle-knife therapy.

It is said that FSN therapy may not work properly if the painful limbs are swelling, or if the pain occurs only in some special position (positional pain), or if there is no clear location of the pain.

(11)   Zhao Wu-Rong Flying acupuncture style (赵武荣飞针针法)

This acupuncture style was developed by Dr. Zhao Wu-Rong and his father.[39] It also depends on meridian diagnosis and TCM diagnosis, as well as the disease local zone selection. The uniqueness of this style is that it works more on meridian as a line or lines, and less on individual acupuncture points. According to the TCM diagnosis, one or more zones or meridians might be stimulated.
The acupuncturist uses needles to stimulate the meridian very quickly without leaving the needle in the points. The needle is mostly inserted only into the skin layer, or under the skin, but not into the muscle. The technique can use a single, ordinary needle, or a bundle of needles (bundle-needle acupuncture).

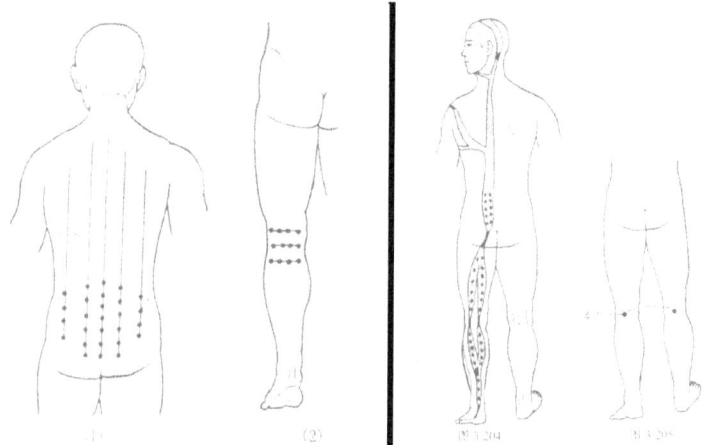

Figure 8. Acupuncture points used by the Flying needle acupuncture style for the treatment of chronic lower back strain.[39]

For example, in the treatment of chronic lumber back strain, the technique uses mass stimulation with needles on the lower back area and the rear part of the knee. It may also use a needle to stimulate the Foot

Taiyang meridian (because this meridian passes through the lower back), plus bleeding therapy on the Weizhong points behind the knee (Figure 8). The treatment can be done once or even twice a day, and at least once every other day.

There are some other similarities to quick acupuncture styles in use in China.[40, 41]

(12)   Li Jin-Niu Five-element acupuncture style (李金牛五行生克针灸)

Traditionally, the original Five-element acupuncture says that each meridian has five acupuncture points that are named after the five elements: Wood, Fire, Soil, Metal, and Water. Also, the 12 body meridians are allocated into one of the five elements. For example, the Heart (small intestine) meridian belongs to Fire, the Spleen (Stomach) meridian belongs to Soil, the Lung (Large intestine) meridian belongs to Metal, the Kidney (Urine bladder) meridian belongs to Water, and the Liver (Gall bladder) meridian belongs to Wood.

The relationship between the elements is as follows: each meridian (and each acupuncture point in the Five element system) gets help from its previous mother meridian (or the mother element point), each nourishes and helps the following meridian (element point) (called son meridian or son point) and each inhibits the grandson meridian (or the grandson element points) that follows the son meridian (or the son element point).

For example, for Liver (Wood) meridian, Kidney (Water) meridian is its mother meridian, Heart meridian (Fire) is its son meridian and the Spleen meridian (Soil) is its grandson meridian. The Liver meridian gets help from the Kidney (Water) meridian, and it helps its son meridian the Heart (Fire) meridian, but counteracts its grandson meridian (the Lung, the Metal meridian). For the five element point in each meridian, this is the same rule.

Traditionally, if any meridian is sick, the acupuncturist can correct the life energy flow in the sick meridian by adjusting the life energy flow in its mother meridian (point) or son meridian (point). If the life energy is overwhelming in the sick meridian, it is necessary to deplete the life energy at the acupuncture point with the same element nature, on its son meridian. If the life energy flow is weak in the sick meridian, it is necessary to nourish the acupuncture point with the same element nature, on its mother meridian.

For example, if the life energy is overwhelming in the Liver meridian, the acupuncturist has two choices: (1) to deplete life energy of the Fire element point on the Liver meridian and (2) to deplete the Fire element on the Fire meridian (the Heart meridian). If the life energy is weak in the Liver meridian, we can also (1) nourish the Water element point on the Liver meridian or (2) nourish the Water element point on the Water (Kidney meridian).

Based on the traditional Five-element acupuncture therapy above, Dr. Li Jin-Niu (2009)[42] further developed modern Five-element acupuncture, taking into the consideration of the reverse-counteract relationship between the five elements.

His idea is that when one element is sick, it will also affect its relationship with other meridians in different ways from those noted above.

If one meridian is overwhelming in life energy flow, it would counteract its grandson meridian (as it normally does), and also reversely counteract its grandmother meridian (normally it is inhibited by its grandmother meridian).

If the life energy flow is weak in one meridian, it would be counteracted by its grandson meridian (which normally is counteracted by the weak meridian), and also be counteracted by its grandmother meridian (normally it has already been counteracted by its grandmother meridian).

For the treatment, if the life energy flow is overwhelming in one meridian, it is necessary to (1) nourish the Element points on the same meridian, which are the same element nature as its grandson meridian and grandmother meridian and (2) nourish the element point on the grandson (grandmother) meridian, which is the same element nature as the grandson (grandmother) meridian.

Let's take an example with the Liver meridian.

If the Life energy flow is overwhelming in the Liver (Wood) meridian, the acupuncturist can either nourish the Spleen point (Taichong) and the Metal point (Zhongfen) on the liver meridian or nourish the Wood point (Taibai) on the Spleen (Wood) meridian and nourish Metal point (Jingqu) on the Lung (Metal) meridian.

If the life energy flow is weak in the Liver (Wood) meridian, the acupuncturist can deplete the Wood point (Taichong) and Metal point

(Zhongfen) on the Liver meridian or deplete the Wood point (Taibai) on the Spleen (Wood) meridian, and deplete the Metal point (Jingqu) on the Lung (Metal) meridian.

For any meridian, follow the same rule.

(13)   Ma Xiao-Ping Five-element acupuncture style (马小平补北泻南法)

This method is another way of using Five-element theory.[43] It said that one element can make its mother element (point or meridian) over-whelming in life energy but weak in life energy in its son element (point or meridian).

For example a Liver-overwhelming-Lung-weakness condition, which is common in clinics,[12] can be treated by depleting Heart (Fire) and nourishing the Kidney (Water) to solve the imbalance. This can be done by depleting the Jing point (the Fire point) while also nourishing the He point (the Water point) on the Heart meridian, or by depleting the Heart meridian (Fire meridian) (or Heart shell meridian, also the Fire meridian), while also nourishing the Kidney meridian (Water meridian).

A similar acupuncture style to this one is the He acupuncture style in Korea.[44]

(14)   Yangming Wuxing acupuncture (阳明五行针法)

This Five-element style is used by Dr. Ding Li-Li[45] for the treatment of obesity. The five element acupuncture points are not the same as the traditional five element points, for which the five element points are on the lower limbs of the 12 meridians (below the elbow and the knee). Its Five-element points are on the whole arm (from shoulder to wrist), whole leg (from hip to ankle), and also on abdomen.

(15)   Mang acupuncture style (蟒针,芒针)

---

[12] Here, the weak lung can be regarded due to the reverse counteract from the overwhelming Liver. Therefore, the aim of the Five-element theory is to reduce the life energy in the Liver side, so as to release the reverse counteraction from the Liver.

Mang needle acupuncture is described in older TCM books[46] but was almost lost for a long time in history in most parts of China. Dr. Wang Shi-Gu learned it from a monk named Shaling, and then expanded on it. Later it was found that it had been used for a long time in a small section of China, known as Yao.

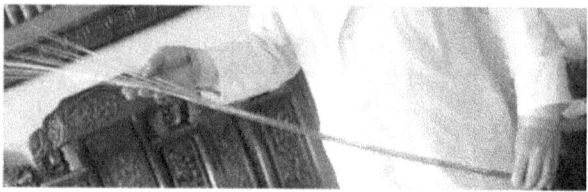

Figure 9. Mang needles. [47]

This acupuncture style follows traditional meridian system,[48, 49, 50] but uses very thick (at least 1 mm in diameter) and very long needles (can be as long as 30 cm or even longer) (Figure 9). It requires very strict disinfection of the needles, the hands of acupuncturist, and the skin. The needle is manipulated under the skin horizontally, and very deeply. The needle is manipulated with either nourishing or deleting techniques. The intensity of the stimulation is said to not be as strong as might be expected. It is also interesting in that it rarely causes bleeding.

(16)   Guo Zhi-Chen Eight-point acupuncture style (郭志辰八穴针法)

This acupuncture style was developed by Dr. Guo Zhi-Chen (1943-2011).[51] It is a supplementary therapy to his Small-formula herbal therapy (草药小方疗法). Both therapies were developed during his Qigong practice. The main idea is that there is big energy in the body, the orbit of the big energy flow is along the middle of the body, from perineal region moving up (in the front of the body) to the top of head, then flowing down through the back of the body, along the spine (the Du meridian), to the perineal region again. It means than the energy flows from the perineal region, along the Ren meridian up to the top of the head, then down along Du meridian to the perineal region.[13] There are

_____

[13] The direction of the major energy flow is different from that of the energy flow in the traditional meridian system, in which the energy flows from perineal

also smaller energies moving horizontally in the body too, but the most important energy flow is the big flow circle.

Diseases can be distributed in either the Upper Jiao cavity (Heart and Lung), the Middle Jiao cavity (Liver, Spleen, Stomach, Intestine), Low Jiao cavity (Kidney, Urine bladder), or Outer Jiao cavity.[14] To maintain the normal energy flow from the Low Jiao, up to the Middle Jiao, to the Upper Jiao, then over the shoulder to the Outer Jiao, or from the Outer Jiao back to the Low Jiao (though the perineal region), it is necessary to clear the front of the sick cavity and to create more energy in the back of the sick cavity, so that we can push the energy flow from the sick cavity further forward to complete the energy circle.

For example, if the disease is in the Upper Jiao, it is necessary to clear the Outer Jiao first, to allow the energy in the Upper Jiao to flow (move) further to front of the Outer Jiao cavity. To enhance the healing, we can also bring more energy from the Middle Jiao cavity to force the energy in the Upper Jiao to move.

Such energy movement therapy can be achieved by using the Small Formula herbal therapy, and also via the eight acupuncture points. The eight acupuncture points are Baihui, Dazhjui, Neiguan, Hegu, Changqiang, Zusanli, Sanyinjiao, and Zhiyin. The eight acupuncture points belong to the traditional acupuncture meridian system, but the function of them in this eight acupuncture style is completely different from traditional acupuncture theory.

According to Dr. Guo, the points Neiguan and Zhiyin work to clear the Upper Jiao, Hegu clears the Middle Jiao, Changqiang and Sanyinjiao clear the Outer Jiao, and Dazhui clears the energy in the head. Baihui moves energy from the top of head to the back of the body (along Du meridian, the Outer Jiao), and Changqiang moves energy from the Outer Jiao (through the perineal region) to the Lower Jiao. Baihui is the upper outlet of extra energy in the three Jiao cavities, and the Zusanli is the lower outlet of the extra energy in the three Jiao cavities.

---

region, along the back of the body – the Du meridian, up to the top of the head, to the upper mouth lip, then down the front the body, along the Ren meridian, to the lower abdomen, then back to the perineal region again.

[14] In the Guo medical system, disease is diagnosed mostly from observation of the tongue.

In this acupuncture style, it is not necessary to get the Deqi sensation.

(17)   Pan Xiao-Chuan Classical acupuncture style (潘晓川古典针灸)

Classical acupuncture style was developed by Dr. Pan Xiao-Chuan.[52] It is different from what is commonly called Traditional acupuncture style. To distinguish this style of acupuncture from the commonly mentioned Traditional acupuncture styles, Dr. Pan named his acupuncture style the Classical acupuncture style.

In this style, the selection of acupuncture points follows meridian, but is based on pulse diagnosis.

For example, if the pulse diagnosis tells us that the heart meridian is weak, the acupuncturist stimulates acupuncture points based on the Primary-Branch relationship of the acupuncture points (原穴络穴), or Five-element theory, etc.

Pan believes that the human body consists of both an energy body (Qi concept in TCM) and a physical body.[53] For a disease, in most cases, the energy body becomes sick before the physical body. The improvement of condition in the physical body can be achieved by improving the energy body.

The aim of the pulse diagnosis is to detect the status of life energy in the body (in each meridian). The pulse acts like a window and is the easiest way to detect the status of life energy in the body. The acupuncture treatment aims to adjust and balance the pulse to a calmed and even level. If the pulse becomes calm, the disease will subside.

Acupuncture can stimulate the flow of the life energy (through feeling on pulse). The energy can be healthy Qi, which feels slow and soft. It can also be an aggressive Qi (disease Qi), which feels fast and aggressive. For a healthy Qi, use the nourishing technique of acupuncture; for the aggressive Qi, use the depleting technique to expel it out of body.

For the pulse, the acupuncturist only needs to identify if the pulse is big or small, deep or floating, slow flowing or fast flowing, and smooth or unsmooth. It is said that it is much simpler than any other currently available pulse diagnosis system.

During treatment, the Deqi sensation is not necessary. Dr. Pan feels that it is strange that the concept of acupuncture treatment depends on Deqi sensation. There is no indication in traditional Chinese medicine books that acupuncture depends on Deqi to exercise its healing effect.

The effective mark for acupuncture treatment is calming of the pulse. If the pulse is not improved (by acupuncture) into a calm status, the disease's symptoms may recur later. If the pulse has been calmed, then the disease would be improved for the long term, even if pain or other discomfort remains and is not corrected yet during the time of the treatment.[15] To get a consistently calm condition of the pulse, a longer time of acupuncture treatment is necessary. It is better to have acupuncture in the morning time and retain the needle for 25 - 30 min.

It should be mentioned that, because the energy flow in the body is believed to be different in the morning and in the afternoon, and that it is also different for male and female, the meanings of the pulse in the left and right wrists are different too.[54] For example, the energy flow for male in the morning is along the left three Yin meridians from chest to the left hand, then along the three Yang meridians from left hand to the upper back, from there along the three Yang meridians to the right hand, then along the three Yin meridians from the right hand to the chest (Figure 10). At the same time, the energy flows along the three Yang meridians in the left leg down to the left foot, along the three Yin meridians in the left leg up to the body trunk, from the body trunk it runs along the three Yin meridians in the right leg down to the right foot, along the three Yang meridians in the right leg up to the body trunk. In the afternoon (from noon), the flow direction is the opposite.

The meaning of the pulse for male in the morning is in the left wrist: Heart (Cun position), Liver (Guan position) and Kidney (Chi position). On the right wrist it is therefore the Lung, Spleen and Life gate. In the afternoon, the pulse in the left wrist becomes Lung, Spleen and Life gate, while the right wrist becomes Heart, Liver and Kidney.

---

[15] It is said that no change in symptoms during treatment does not mean that there is no healing effect yet.

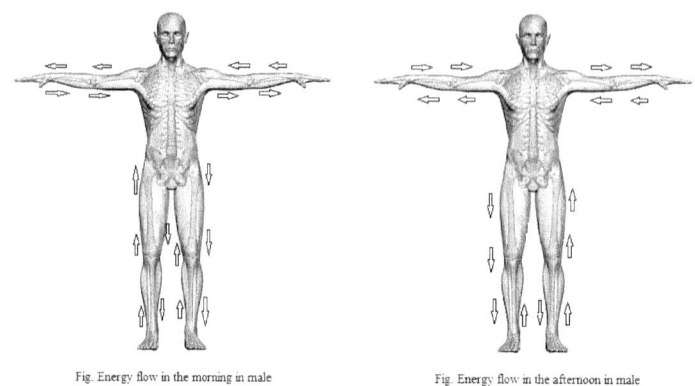

Fig. Energy flow in the morning in male   Fig. Energy flow in the afternoon in male

Figure 10. Energy flow direction in the morning and afternoon in male.

For female, the flow direction is opposite of the male in both morning and afternoon.

(18)   Korea Sha-Am Five-element acupuncture (韩国舍岩五行针法)

This Five-element acupuncture style [55] also came from China, but was developed and applied more by Korea acupuncturists. There are some similarities between the Sha-am acupuncture style and the Five-element introduced above. For the purpose of this article, we omit the details of application.

(19)   Korea Li Ji-Ma Four-diagram acupuncture style (李济马太极四象针灸)

The Tai-Ji Four-diagram acupuncture (李济马太极四象针灸) was developed by Dr. Li Ji-Ma and later further developed by Dr. Li Bing-Xin (李炳幸) in Korea.[56] This style of acupuncture diagnoses the body condition of a patient into four kinds: Taiyang, Taiyin, Shaoyang and Shaoyin. For the Taiyang, the Lung is stronger and the Liver is weaker. For Taiyin, the Liver is stronger and the Lung is weaker. For Shaoyang, the Spleen is stronger and the Kidney is weaker. For Shaoyin, the Kidney is stronger and the Spleen is weaker.

For the treatment, we use the Five Shu points in the Heart meridian and take into consideration the Five-element nature of the five points. The style also uses the Primary points of the traditional meridians for the treatment, based on the Five-element theory.

(20)   Nora Five-element acupuncture style (Nora 五行针法)

Nora Five-element acupuncture style [57] originated in China a long time ago. It was discontinued for a long time in China but survived in Korea and Japan. Later it was re-developed in England by J. R. Worsley and Nora Franglen.

This Five-element acupuncture style separates humans into five elements. Any person has one element that dominates his or her physical body function and emotional status. The dominant element stays with the person forever. Disease or symptoms cause an imbalance of the elements. The doctor needs to find out the dominant element of the patient and restore it via acupuncture treatment. To find out the dominant element of the patient, the acupuncturist needs to collect information from the four major aspects of the patient: voice, color, smell/odor and emotional status. The acupuncturist also needs to collect other, broader information about the patient such as life style and emotional relationship with others. We need a very close relationship between the doctor and the patient to get sufficient and correct physical and emotional information about the patient.[58] It is therefore claimed that this acupuncture style is not only able to treat the physical illness but also to improve the emotions of patients.

For pulse diagnosis, it is admitted that it cannot be used to help find the dominant element for the patient, but it can find the pulse indicating a poor relationship between husband and wife, and the pulse indicating energy flow blockage in the connection with two meridians.[59]

The acupuncturist also touches the body (the chest, the upper abdomen and lower abdomen) to find any imbalance within the Three Jiao, presses the Mu point to find any imbalance in each organ, and to touches the middle vertical line of the abdomen to find position changes of the abdominal aorta.[16]

The acupuncturist also uses the Akabane test[17] to find energy flow imbalances in the Jing points (the acupuncture points that are located on the fingers or toes) between the left and the right side of the body. If there is an imbalance, we must do acupuncture on the weak side of Jing point (using nourishing technique). Then we must test it again. If the imbalance remains, we do acupuncture on the Origin point of the meridian on the stronger side (also using nourishing technique). This treatment procedure needs to be repeated several times until the warm sensation on the Jing points on both sides of the body becomes equal.

After set up of the element diagnosis, the treatment might be relatively simple, because each element body has its own specific and co-related acupuncture points to stimulate. The whole treatment course is separated into different phases. Each phase has its own specific treatment goal. In the beginning, the acupuncturist mildly stimulates the 12 meridians. It works almost as a test period to see if the diagnosis of the dominant element is correct or not.

Here is an example for the treatment:

If a patient is diagnosed as Element Metal, on the first treatment, the acupuncturist will do acupuncture on Hegu and Taiyuan (both are the Primary point of the Lung meridian).

During the second treatment, the acupuncturist uses point Jingqu (to clear the garbage on the Lung meridian), Wood point Quchi and Taiyuan (to nourish the Lung meridian: mother meridian to nourish the son meridian: using Quchi and Taiyuan), Fire point (Fire counteract the

---

[16] If there is position change with the abdominal aorta, the acupuncturist uses his hand to correct it.

[17] Akabane test: test the warm sensation of each Jing point on fingers and toes (total 12 such points) to see if the warm sensation on the Jing points on the left and right hands, and the left and right feet, are the same or not. If the sensation on one side is different from other side, it indicates imbalance of Qi flow between the two points. Use a burned line moxi to move close to the point and ask the patient if the patient feels warm at the point. The acupuncturist makes a record of how many times the patient starts to feel warm after the burned moxi moves over a spot. Most of time, the Jing points on the feet need about 10-20 times to feel warm and the Jing points on the hands need about 3-10 times.

Metal, using point Yuji), and Wood point (using Taiyuan, Yinbai, Yuji, or Zhongchong).

During the third treatment, the patient complains of some discomfort, poor digestion, and stiffness in the sinuses. It is found from pulse diagnosis that the pulse on the Metal is stronger than the Wood, indicating an energy flow block in the large intestine and stomach. The acupuncturist uses point Yingxiang and Chengqi to remove the block. After removal of the block, it is necessary to decide if the treatment needs to use Primary point, or some other points, to improve energy flow in the meridians.

During the forth treatment, the patient feels a little better overall, but still feels depression. Acupuncture is performed on the Shenque point (Use moxi only. If there is hypertension, use Juque point only.). Again, it is necessary to decide if the treatment needs to use Primary point or some other points to improve energy flow in the meridians.

During the fifth treatment, use corresponding body back Shu point to the Metal, the Large intestine Shu point and the Lung Shu point. After treatment, again it is necessary to decide if the treatment needs to use Primary point or some other points to improve energy flow in the meridians.

It is emphasized that if the treatment above is performed in the fall, it is necessary to also use the Season point once. For Metal, the Season points are Shangyang (the Metal point on the Large intestine meridian) and the Jingqu point (the Metal point on the Lung meridian). These use the universe's energy to nourish the body energy.

During treatment, the body condition of the patient can show more clearly whether the person belongs to the Metal element. If so, the treatment can go further into the next phase. If it is not clear yet, the above treatment procedure has to be repeated to test for other Elements.

For the following treatment phase, the acupuncturist performs acupuncture on points that belong to the Metal meridian. Based on body condition, some points on the other meridians may also be stimulated, such as points on the body back (Urine bladder meridian), Du meridian and Ren meridian.

In the Five-element acupuncture style, we emphasize the use of Season circle and Daily circle of the energy flow in the meridians. It requires Deqi sensation. For nourishing technique, the needle is removed after getting the Deqi sensation. For depleting technique, the needle remains in spot for 20 min. Overall, the needle is inserted shallower than most of other acupuncture styles.

For such a treatment plan, we need at least 8-10 sessions of treatment. Acupuncturists in this style do not emphasize the importance of each acupuncture point. They tend not to stimulate the patient with a large number of acupuncture points, nor with stronger stimulation, so as to prevent the disturbance to the energy flow in the body. They do not aim to get quick improvement. They do not know what may happen next with their treatment, because each patient is different and the reaction of patient to the treatment is also very complex. It is claimed that the highest goal for such treatment is to change the life of the patient.

For treatment frequency, acupuncture is usually performed once per week. Once there is a sign of clear and constant improvement, acupuncture sessions can be changed to once every ten days, then once every two weeks, then once every two months.

(a). Aggressive Energy: This style also pays attention to the treatment of Aggressive energy (AE). Removal of the AE is the basic work before applying the typical Five-element therapy. We use the body back Shu points for the treatment.[18] According to Five-element theory, the AE passes from the mother meridian to the son (counteracting the relationship between meridians). Without stopping its pass, the AE will damage all the meridians. To remove the AE, use the following body back Shu points: Heart Shell Shu, Liver Shu, Spleen Shu, Lung Shu, Kidney Shu.[19] The needles should be inserted shallowly and also at an oblique angle. If indeed there is AE in the body, there will be a pink color around these needles. It is necessary to wait and not to pull out the needles until the skin color disappears.[20]

(b). Attached energy body: the patient is affected by an extra energy body. The patient who is affected by the extra spirit body may behave

---

[18] Other acupuncture systems may use Five Shu points to removal the AE out of body.

[19] Heart Shu is used only when there is AE in the heart.

[20] It may take 20 min to 2 hours. But if the pink color does not disappear after some time, it may not mean that there is AE in the body. However, our own experience is that if there is pink color around needles on the back of the body, the healing effect of acupuncture is very good. We do not regard it as aggressive energy; it means that the body is sensitive to acupuncture stimulation.

strangely. In severe cases, the patient may appear to have a mental disease. For the treatment, the acupuncturist uses Inner-Seven-Dragon points: Jiuwei, Tianshu, Futu, and Jiexi. If the treatment does not work, the acupuncturist uses Outside-Seven-Dragon points: Baihui, Dazhu, Shenshu and Pucan.

(c). Imbalance of left-right pulse: if the pulse on the left side (called the husband side) is weaker than that on the right side (called wife side), there is a Wife-Husband imbalance.[21] For the treatment, we transfer the energy from the right side to the left side using the Five-element theory and the Primary-point theory.

(d). Meridian energy flow block: the energy flow is blocked from one meridian to next. The block happens mostly in the area where the two meridians connect. Such blocks can only be diagnosed by pulse, or by some physical illness sign around the blocked area. The most severe block is the block between the Du meridian and the Ren meridian, showing as weak pulse on both hands. For treatment, nourish the outlet point of the first meridian and the inlet point of the following meridian (both with nourishing technique).

(e). Scar tissue. Scar tissue could block the energy flow through meridian. For treatment, the acupuncturist stimulates the points located on both side of the scar tissue, with nourishing technique.

It is said that the treatment starts when the acupuncturist meets the patient and starts to have communication, not only from the use of needles. We can predict that this style needs a longer time to correct disorders of the body. Along with treatment (and personal relationship), the acupuncturist may change his diagnosis again and again. This style might be regarded more as emotional re-balance. Physical disorders can be corrected through the improvement of emotional/spiritual aspects.

We have not practiced this Five-element acupuncture yet, but we have concerns about it:

(a) It requires the acupuncturist to have good communication skills to talk with patients, and requires the acupuncturist to communicate the way that the patient prefers.

---

[21] It may not really mean the poor relationship between the husband and his wife.

(b) It might be too simple to separate human beings into only the five elements, because, as we understand, the body elements of most people is a mixture of two or three or even more types of elements. For example, a person's body element might be mixture of Wood and Fire constitution, or Metal and Water elements. For a mixed body constitution, one element might be more dominant than another.

(c) It would be difficult to get correct information for elemental diagnosis if the patient refuses to reveal his or her personal information.[58, 60]

(d) The acupuncturist needs to keep his or her own emotions in a balanced and have a peaceful status (as a mirror), so as to be sensitive enough to understand the emotional status of the patient.

(e) What if the acupuncturist's own dominant elements are Metal and Water? [22]

(f) We might spend unnecessary time on patients if the patient only wants to stop the pain as soon as possible.

Because this Five-element acupuncture style has greater emphasis on communication with patients, it seems more dependent on the psychological aspect of the treatment. The healing effect might be relatively more depending on a psychological effect, which might be doubted as a placebo effect.

It might be difficult to test if this Five-element acupuncture style is mostly dependent on a placebo effect, given current strategies of acupuncture research in Western countries, in which communication between acupuncturist and patient is restricted. Without communication

---

[22] Theoretically, Element Metal shows as cool, and inner-forwarded, and people are not good at social communication but are good at job techniques. Element Water is quiet (as winter), and such people are also not good at social communication. During communication with patients, doctors who practice the Five-element therapy need to meet the needs of patients to know the doctor's personal information. A Metal and Water element doctor might be hesitant to share such personal information with patients. So, we predict that the proper element of a doctor who participates in such Five-element might best be Fire - Wood - Soil - Metal - Water combined. But, even so, if the patient is of the Water element, he or she might not like to meet a doctor who is too warm (a Fire element doctor). The co-relationship between the element of the doctor and that of the patient is important.

between the acupuncturist and patient, how could the Five-elements of this style of acupuncture work? Currently, we can only find someone exploring the theoretical possibility to use this style of acupuncture to treat post-stroke depression patients.[61] Such a study might be difficult since patients are usually hesitant to communicate.

Overall, we feel that this type of so-called Five-element acupuncture is not an individual acupuncture style, but mixes acupuncture methods in the practical environment of an acupuncture clinic.

Knowing the dominant element of patients seems to have nothing to do with the treatment of their physical illness. The healing effect of this style of acupuncture can be attributed to various acupuncture methods used during treatment: (1) during the Akabane test, the moxi used has stimulated the acupuncture points (the Jing points of all the 12 meridian); (2) continuous stimulation of the Primary acupuncture points during different steps of the treatment; (3) in the release of block due to scar tissue; (4) in the treatment of aggressive Energy; (5) in the treatment of the attached energy body; (6) in the use of Spiritual Window points (to open the heart/emotion of a patient to the outside environment/world); (7) routine use of moxibustion before every needle stimulation; (8) frequent use of the Primary points during every treatment step.

In all of these treatment courses, the acupuncturist does not apply the Five-element theory for the treatment.

Once coming into Five-element therapy, it seems that the acupuncturist only believes that the principle problem for every patient is that his dominant element is weak and the dominant Element needs to be nourished. Therefore, the nourishing technique is principally used, which includes non-retention of the needle in the acupuncture point (if the needle is left for 20 to 30 min, it is regarded as a depleting technique).

If so, it seems that the acupuncturist does not follow the typical principle for the use of the Five-element theory. In typical Five-element acupuncture styles, in the case of the deficient Element/meridian, the meridian condition should be corrected by stimulating its mother Element. If the meridian is in an overwhelming status, we need to stimulate its son Element/meridian. At the same time, the Element or the meridian that resists the sick meridian, should not be stimulated because to stimulate this resisting meridian would make the sick Element/meridian weaker (one of the reasons for its weakness is due to suppression from another Element/meridian).

An example is given: the patient's body Element is diagnosed as Metal. It said that all of the treatment should be with a nourishing technique to support the Metal meridian (the Lung meridian and the Large intestine meridian). This means that the acupuncturist believes that the energy in the Lung meridian and the Large intestine meridian is weak.

In the first treatment, the acupuncture points Taiyuan and Hegu are used. The point Taiyuan is the Soil point in the Lung meridian. This is a correct use, according to Chinese Five-element theory, but the point Hegu is the Fire point in the Large intestine meridian. The Fire suppresses the Metal, so the use of Hegu may not be a proper choice. The acupuncturist uses it just because it is the Primary point of the Large intestine meridian. It seems that the primary point can be used at any time, without need to consider its element nature in this style of acupuncture.

From the second treatment, they emphasize the use of other acupuncture points to connect the life energy from other meridians to the Metal meridian. The points used are:

(a) Quchi and Taiyuan. The use of Taiyuan is fine because it is the Wood point in the Metal meridian. The use of Quchi is also fine, because it is the Wood point in the Large intestine meridian. The Wood point/meridian is the mother of the Metal point/meridian and it nourishes the Metal;

(b) Yuji. The Yuji point is the Fire point in the Lung meridian. It is not a proper point because the Fire suppresses the Metal;

(c) Yinbai or Zhongchong. The Yinbai point is the Wood point in the Spleen meridian (Wood meridian). Normally the Metal point/meridian suppresses the Wood. If the Metal is weak, the Wood would be able to suppress Metal in turn, especially if we stimulate the Wood to make it stronger. This is not a good acupuncture point choice. It is better to use the Taibai (Wood point) in the Spleen meridian (Wood meridian). The Wood nourishes the Metal. The Zhongchong is the Soil point in the Liver meridian (Wood meridian). It is hard to understand what would be the result of stimulating the Soil point in the Wood meridian on the energy status in the Metal.

Five-element is already complex for most of beginners in acupuncture. The use of the Five-elements in this style of acupuncture seems even more complex and difficult to understand according to traditional Five-element theory. According to the author, they use, at the same time, both the assistance relationship between the mother point/meridian (相生) and the son point/meridian, and the resistance relationship between the given point/meridian and its grandmother point/meridian (相克). They use the Yin and Yang points in either meridian to balance the life energy among the meridians. The idea is that, when the dominant meridian is weak, the acupuncturist can transfer energy from other meridians to support it. Once the energy is sufficient in the dominant meridian, it would likely and willingly share its energy with other meridians too.

It is also strange that the acupuncturist refuses to stimulate the acupuncture points on the Heart meridian, for the worry that it may otherwise disturb the emotion and spirit of the patient. This is absolutely unaccepted by the traditional Chinese acupuncture community. One of the Korean acupuncture styles also separates the body into Elements, but uses the Five element points in the Heart meridian to correct the imbalance among the four elements of the body.

We also ask why acupuncture always starts from the left side of the body.

Acupuncturists in this acupuncture style emphasize having a long treatment schedule. They believe that the whole treatment needs a long time to complete, and they do not expect quick improvement of body condition with their treatment. They worry that acupuncture stimulation may disturb the Qi and Blood environment of patients, so they recommend using the least possible number of needles, and have the fewest possible treatments. They cannot expect or predict what may happen to the patients with their treatment because they feel that each patient is different in the reaction to the treatment. However, they still claim that the highest goal of the treatment is to help the patient change their life.

This type of Five-element acupuncture is mostly practiced by acupuncturists in the UK, where there are several acupuncture schools that teach it.

(21)   Japanese acupuncture

There are many different acupuncture systems in Japan.[62] One of the interesting characteristics of acupuncture in Japan is that some acupuncturists do not pay attention to the meridian diagnosis, and use the abdomen touching diagnosis instead. They find the painful spot in the abdomen (the A Shi point) and stimulate it during treatment. They insert the needles at a very shallow angle. Needles are very thin and they use large number. Deqi sensation is sought.[63]

One style of Japanese acupuncture is the Japanese Meridian acupuncture system (Keiraku Chiryo).[64, 65] It emphasizes the diagnosis using the pulse on the wrist. It is believed that the imbalance in the distribution of the Qi in the meridians is the cause of disease. Stimulation of the meridian could restore the normal distribution and circulation of the life Qi in the meridians. They also use acupuncture needles, but the needles are inserted very shallowly (1- 2 mm, or not even penetrating the skin). They do not aim to induce the Deqi sensation and the patient does not feel anything, or only feels a very mild stimulation. However, they emphasize that the acupuncturist should feel the energy in the meridians.

Another Japanese acupuncture style is the Kiiko Matsumoto Japanese Style,[66] which is currently available in US. It emphasizes the use of palpation on the abdomen to find the reason for a disease. In the treatment, the needle insertion is very shallow.

(22)   Various special manipulating techniques of acupuncture

There are also some more acupuncture styles that are used mostly in China. They usually choose acupuncture points from the traditional meridians but use a special way of manipulating needles for better treatment results. Examples for such special acupuncture are as follows:

Xing Nao Kai Qiao method by Dr. Shi Xue-Min (石学敏醒脑开窍针刺法);[67,68]
Fei Jing Zou Qi method by Dr. Zhen Kui-Shan, Li Yu-Lin, Lu Shou-Kang, and Wang Fu-Chun (郑魁山, 李毓麟, 陆寿康, 王富春之各种飞经走气法);[69,70,71,72,73,74]
Big Meridian-connecting method by Dr. Zhang Yuan-Su (张元素大接经法);[75]

Governor Vessel-regulating and brain-unblocking acupuncture method by Dr. Gao Yu-Pei and his father Dr. Gao Yu-Chun (调督通脑针刺法);[76]
Target acupuncture by Dr. He Tian-You (何天有靶向针刺法);[77]
Tong Luo An Shen by Dr. Li Ming-Yue (李明月通络安神针刺法);[78]
Yi Shen Tong Qiao by Dr. Yu Chuan (于川益肾通窍针法);[79]
Tian Kun acupuncture method by Dr. Li Ji-Chun (李济春乾坤针法);[80]
Lifting and pressing method by Dr. Ding Bang-You (丁邦友抽添针灸疗法);[81]
Tong Du Tiao Shen acupuncture method by Dr. Li Ping (李平通督调神针法);[82]
Shallow stimulating acupuncture techniques (各种皮下浅刺法[(23)]);[83,84,85,86]
Motivating-tendon acupuncture by Dr. Chen De-Cheng (陈德成动筋针法);[87]
Nou Yun Zhi Zhen acupuncture by Dr. Lou Mei (路玫努运滞针法);[88]
Zhu Tong Yi Ten acupuncture by Dr. Wen Hong (文洪教授 "住痛移疼" 针法);[89]
Around acupuncture technique (围刺法).[90]

2. Acupuncture styles only partly following traditional meridian

(1) Dong Jing-Chang extraordinary point acupuncture style (董氏奇穴疗法)

This style of acupuncture[91] was developed by Dr. Dong Jing-Chang (1916-1975). Later it was further developed by his students Yang Wei-Jie, Hu Wen-Zhi, Li Guo-Zhi and others.

The acupuncture points are distributed all over the body, but in most cases the points do not follow the traditional meridians. Instead, the distribution and the selection of the acupuncture points partially follow the Holographic theory.

Holographic theory (全息理论) states that any one part of the body contains the information about the whole body. Therefore, stimulation on a local spot can influence the co-related part of the whole body. For example, one front arm can be regarded as the whole (small) body. If the far-end (e.g. the wrist) part of the arm represents the head of the whole

---

[(23)] Mostly in the dermis layer, e.g. 2-3 mm from surface of skin, aimed to have Deqi sensation. If the needle is in the hypodermis, there is no aim to induce the Deqi sensation.

body, the near-end (e.g. the elbow part) of the arm would represent the foot of the whole body. If a person has pain on their foot, we can choose acupuncture points (belonging to meridians or not) near the wrist.

This style of acupuncture also partially follows a Mirror theory (镜像理论). This means that one part of the body can be regarded as a mirror part of another part of the body. For example, the head and foot have a mirror relationship. If a person has a headache, we can stimulate acupuncture points (also on the meridian or not) on the foot. If a person has pain on their left hand, we can perform acupuncture on the right hand (on a similar pain spot) or on the right foot too. Here the left hand and right hand have a mirror relationship, as do the left hand and the right foot.

Five-shu theory (五腧穴理论).

In this style of acupuncture, the acupuncture points are selected and based on the function of five Shu points on the 12 meridians. For example, for all the Jing points,[24] they can be used to treat stroke and other brain diseases (especially for acute diseases), or to treat bloating in the abdomen.

This style of acupuncture also has a special Five-element system (五行理论). Many of the acupuncture points are directly named as either Wood, Fire, Soil, Metal or Water, or in combination, such as Wood point, Fire-lian point, Wood-Fire point, and Soil-Metal point. The five elements can be distributed on a line, such as the Minghuang, Tianhuang and Qihuang (inside of thigh), all of which belong to Liver (the Wood line), or the Tianhuang, Renhuang, Dihuang (in the inside of calf), which belong to Kidney (Water line). The five elements can also be distributed as a zone in the body, such as the Fire zone, Metal zone, Soil zone and Wood zone on the upper back, or the Fire zone and Water zone,on the feet. From the name, acupuncturist should be able to realize what kind of disease these acupuncture points can work for.

The Five-element usage in this style of acupuncture is one of the greatest contributions to the Chinese acupuncture system.

---

[24] Each of the 12 traditional meridian systems has one its own Jing point, which is believed to be the beginning of life energy in each meridian.

Organ-bypass theory.

Additionally, acupuncture point selection follows Organ-organ bypass theory (脏腑别通). This theory states that life energy can also flow to other specific meridians that do not belong to the Surface-inside relationship (for example, the Gall bladder meridian and the Liver meridian have a Surface-inside relationship). In the Organ-organ bypass theory, for example, the Large intestine meridian is not connected (by-passed) to the Liver meridian.[25] This can explain how several acupuncture points on or close to the hand Yangming meridian (such as Dajian, Xiaojian, Waijian, Fujian points) can be used to treat diseases in testicle, hernia, urethritis and the perineum area. This is because the Liver meridian passes and goes around the perineum. It is said that the function of at least one third of the acupuncture points in this style can be explained with the Organ-organ bypass theory.[92]

Structure-corresponding structure theory (体体相应).

This theory states that we can stimulate a tendon to treat tendon-related diseases, stimulate bone membrane (bone) to treat bone-related diseases, stimulate muscle to treat muscle-related diseases, stimulate skin to treat skin disorders.

Structure-corresponding phase theory (体象相应).

This theory states that the stimulation of a tendon can treat Wind disease, the stimulation of muscle can treat Wetness, stimulation of bone (membrane) can treat Cold disease, etc.

Depth-effect theory (深度效应).

It is believed that on a given acupuncture point, shallow needles work for shallow diseases (such as disease on the skin, or on the upper part of the body) and nearby diseases. Deeper needles work for distant diseases or inner organ diseases. For example to perform acupuncture on the Zusanli point, shallow needles treat diseases on leg, middle-deep

---

[25] In the bypass theory, Yangming meridian connects with Jueyin meridian; Taiyang meridian connects with Taiyin meridian; and Shaoyang meridian connects with Shaoyin meridian.

needles work for diseases in the stomach-intestine, and deep needles work for diseases in the heart and lung. For facial paralysis, the needle has to be 2 cun deep and with needle tip pointing towards the head.

In this style, we do not emphasize the nourishing-depleting technique of the needle. Instead, we may apply two or more needles close together (in special sequence), for example in what they call the reverse-horse needle technique to enhance the healing effect. We can also apply the moving technique to enhance the healing effect. The style also uses penetrating needle (e.g. one needle penetrates two or more acupuncture points), such as from Linggu point to Dabai point.

This is a very complex and comprehensive acupuncture style.

(2) Ke Shang-Zhi Distance-meridian acupressure therapy (柯尚志远络疗法)

Distance-meridian acupressure therapy was developed by Dr. Ke Shang-Zhi.[93] It only partially follows the traditional Chinese meridian theory. For this technique, we need to find the diseased (sick) meridian first, and then decide which will be the treating meridians. There are three meridians used usually to balance the sick meridian: the same name meridian,[26] the bypass meridian, and the surface-inner relationship meridian.

For example, if the sick meridian is the Hand Yangming meridian, the treatment meridian by the same name would be the Foot Yangming meridian. For the bypass meridian, the treatment meridian would be the Foot Yueyin meridian. And for the surface-inner relationship meridian, the treatment meridian would be the Hand Taiyin meridian on the other arm.

After identifying the sick meridian, the acupuncturist presses the Luo point on the meridian with a finger or with something hard, pressing tightly against the bone under it. At the same time, the acupuncturist

---

[26] There are differences in how to decide the same-name meridian in traditional Chinese meridian theory and this distance-meridian therapy. In the former, the three Hands Yang meridians match the three Foot Yang meridians and the three Hand Yin meridians match the three Foot Yin meridians. In this distance-meridian therapy, the three Hand Yang meridians also match the three Foot Yang meridian, but the Hand Taiyin (lung) matches Foot Jueyin (liver), Hand Jueyin (Heart shell) matches Foot Shaoyin (Kidney), and Hand Shaoyin (Heart) matches Foot Taiyin (Spleen) meridian.

presses the treating point on each of the treating meridians with either nourishing technique (press and moving along the flow direction of the life energy in the meridian) or depleting technique (press the treating point towards the opposite direction of the life energy flow in that meridian, with the speed of the patient's heart beats).[27] Therefore, this is a two- point acupressure technique.[28]

The Luo point is claimed to open the connection of energy flow between the sick meridian and the three treating meridians (traditionally it only connects with the other meridian that has a surface-inner relationship to the sick meridian). There are 14 Luo points in this style, not the traditional 15 Luo points. Among the 14 Luo points, only 4 Luo points are in the same position as in the traditional acupuncture meridian system.[94] The Luo point on the sick meridian needs to press hard against the bone without movement.

Treatment points on the other meridians can be found and decided according to parallel-mimic theory of the Holographic theory. This theory means that information on a whole arm is equal to a whole leg, or to that in the trunk of the body (Figure 11). The arm, the leg, or the body trunk is separated into zones a, b, c, and 1 to 6. The wrist and the ankle are the separating line, marked as a. The hands and foot are b and c. Over the wrist and ankle are separated into 1 to 6. According to the pain spot on the sick meridian, it is necessary to find the treatment spot on the treatment meridians in the corresponding zone.

If the patient fears the pain pressing, the Luo point and the treatment points can be stimulated by finger (or by acupuncture needle).

Though it has been claimed that this style of acupuncture can eliminate the pain of various disorders,[95] it has also been pointed out by others[96] that it works mostly for functional disorders, such as various traumas, chronic pain (in the shoulder, neck, back, limbs), dizziness, migraines, and lingering pain after Herpes Zoster. It does not work properly for structural disorders, such as carpel channel syndrome, trigger finger, frozen shoulder, or sciatica pain due to piriformis syndrome. If the pain

---

[27] If the treatment meridian is the Yin meridian, press the meridian that is opposite to the sick meridian (except for the Liver meridian). If it is the Yang meridian, press the meridian that is on the same side of the sick meridian (except for the Heart meridian).
[28] Two-point treatment technique can also be found in the Moving acupuncture technique in Dong's extra-ordinary acupuncture system.

is due to a structural disorder, the passive movement of the body part would be restricted and limited, or the pain comes and goes after the distance-meridian therapy treatment. In this case, it is recommended to use small knife-needle therapy for treatment.[29] The clinical efficiency of the Distance-meridian therapy has been tested, but with acupuncture on traditional Luo pints and needle stimulation, not with acupressure or with hard materials.[97]

It has also been summarized that this style of acupuncture may not work properly in the following conditions:

(a) If a disease is in central nerve system, this acupressure technique does not work as well if the pain is caused by local damage to muscle or tendon. Knowledge of Western medicine is needed to identify if the pain is due to local or to central nerve system.

(b) If the Five-element nature of the sick meridian is the same as the nature of the seasons, the healing effect might be low. For example, if the sick meridian is the Gall bladder meridian, then the Wood meridian, the treatment meridian for the sick Gall bladder meridian (as well as the Liver meridian) would be hard in spring. Similarly, the Fire nature meridian (the Heart meridian and Small intestine meridian) would be hard to improve in summer (Summer belongs to Fire). The Water nature meridian (Kidney meridian and Urine bladder meridian) would be hard to improve in winter (winter belongs to Water). The Soil nature meridian (the Spleen meridian and Stomach meridian) would be hard to improve in June, July and August (these three months belong to Soil element).

(c) Acute pain would re-occur more readily than chronic pain. Pain in younger patients is easier to re-occur than in elderly patients.

(d) If the local inflammation is severe, then the inflammation needs to be under control before using this acupressure technique for the treatment.

The major weakness for this style of acupuncture is the pain that is created by acupuncturist when the acupuncturist presses the Luo point and the treatment points, though some people claimed that the technique does not touch the original pain spot of the body. The users of this style

---

[29] But proponents of distance-acupressure therapy claims that the advantage of using it is to not touch the painful spot causing local damage.

of acupuncture also claim that this technique is the combination of knowledge from both Chinese medicine and Western medicine. Difficulties arise if the acupuncturist does not have knowledge of Western medicine to find out, and to choose, the Luo points and the treatment points for the treatment.[30] As pointed out above, this technique does not work properly if the Five-element nature of the sick meridian and that of the season is the same (even if the developer of this style of acupuncture claimed that he had found new explanation and new usage of the Five-element theory). For example if the patient suffers from sick Liver meridian and the patient comes for treatment in Spring, the healing effect might not be good.

Overall, it seems that this style of acupuncture works more as a short-term pain killer. It may surprise the patient with its quick pain-reduction effect (for some kinds of pain), but may create new troubles in the future for the acupuncture as a whole. If so, patients may be hesitant to come back again, just because they could use a regular pain killer, which does not create more pain during treatment as this technique does.

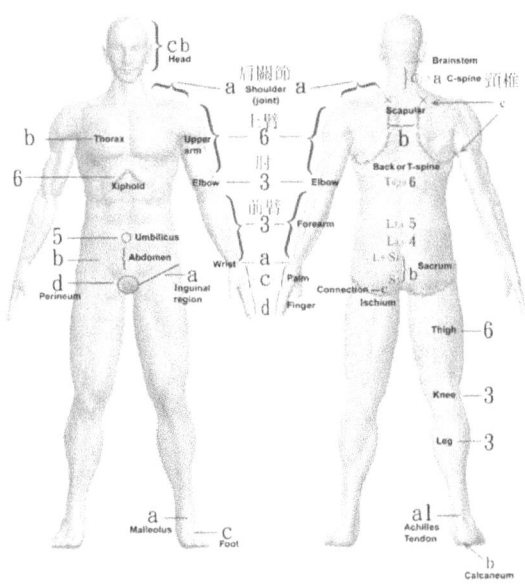

---

[30] Dr. Ke also explained how our body feels pain, with his rich knowledge in Pathophysiology in Western medicine. It is difficult for us to understand the usefulness of such knowledge in using this technique for the treatment.

Figure 11. Mirror distribution and location of pain spots and treating zone in Ke Shang-Zhi Distance-meridian acupressure therapy.[98]

There are some similarities between this acupressure technique and the Li Bai-Son Eight-word acupuncture style (李柏松八字疗法). In this acupressure style, the Luo points are pressed hard against the bone, and in the latter, the bone membrane is stimulated with needles. Both stimulate the bone membrane very strongly.

(3) Han Wen-Zhi One-needle Acupuncture style (韩文治一针疗法)

This acupuncture style was developed by Dr. Han Wen-zhi (Taiwan). [99] This style is very different from traditional acupuncture style. It has its own meridian system, called Qi-Jing-Liu-Mai (e.g. extraordinary meridian and six meridian systems). The meridians are called Heart-Lung meridian, Liver-Gall-bladder meridian, Spleen-Stomach meridian, Large-Intestine-Small-Intestine meridian, and Kidney-Du-Ren meridian. The locations of these meridians and the spot or connections between two meridians are also very different from the traditional meridian system. Beside this difference, there are 14 special acupuncture points in use (though some points belong to the traditional acupuncture system too).

Basically, each treatment session uses only one acupuncture point. Needles are inserted slowly. Acupuncture techniques of nourishing or depleting are needed. Deqi is needed. The needle is usually retained for 20-30 min, with manipulation from time to time.

There are another 12 special acupuncture points in use, which are named after the commonly used 12 animal signs for birth years in China: the mouse point, cow point, tiger point, rabbit point, snake point, horse point, sheep point, etc. For most of these points, the needles are inserted as deep as 2 to 3 body cun, but one needle is used only.[100] For the treatment of some special diseases, more needles are used the same time, such as for the treatment of hypertension.[101]

(4) Zhang Xin-Shu wrist-ankle acupuncture style (腕踝针法)

Wrist-ankle acupuncture style was developed by Prof. Zhang Xin-Shu in year 1972.[102] In this style, needles are inserted in a spot on the front arm 2 finger lengths[31] from the wrist, or 3 finger lengths from the ankle. There are six spots on each front arm and also six spots on each shin (Figure 12). The arm and leg are separated into six zones (Figure 13). Each spot responds for the treatment of disease that are located in that zone. For example, if there is pain on the leg, which is located in zone A, the acupuncturist can stimulate the acupuncture spot that works for that zone. In this style, we prevented any feeling of the needle. If the patient feels pain, or tingling, or bloating, the healing effect would be lower than if the patient feels nothing.

For diseases that are located above the diaphragm, use points on wrist. If the disease is in the wrist or hand, the tips of the needles point towards the hand. Otherwise, point towards the shoulder direction.

If the disease is located below the diaphragm, use the points on the ankle. If the disease is on the ankle or foot, the tips of the needles point towards the feet. Otherwise they point towards the hip.

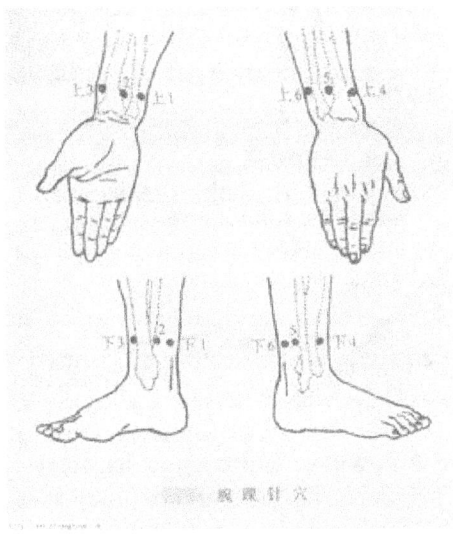

Figure 12. Acupuncture points used in the Wrist-ankle acupuncture style.[103]

If the disease is in both upper and lower part of the body, choose the acupuncture points on both wrist and on ankle, such as for the treat-

---

[31] Cun is a Chinese medicine way of measure length. One cun equals one inch.

ment of paralysis. If it is hard to decide which side the disease is, such as with depression or poor sleep, use both sides.

All the treatment zones are vertically distributed on the body, either from hands to the chest, or from the feet to the body trunk (Figure 13).

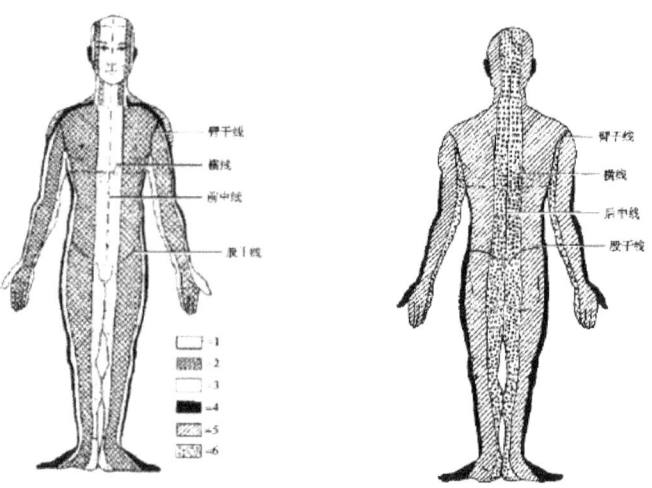

Front zones of Wrist-ankle acupuncture   Rear zones of Wrist-ankle acupuncture

Figure 13. Front zones and rear zones of Wrist-ankle acupuncture style.[104]

(5) Western style of Medicine Acupuncture

Finally we have to mention a modified style of acupuncture that is used mostly in Western countries.

White, A. (2009)[105] introduced the following: Western medical acupuncture is a therapeutic modality involving the insertion of fine needles. It is an adaptation of Chinese acupuncture using current knowledge of anatomy, physiology and pathology, and the principles of evidence based medicine. While Western medical acupuncture has evolved from Chinese acupuncture, its practitioners no longer adhere to concepts such as *Yin/Yang* and circulation of *qi*, and regard acupuncture as part of conventional medicine rather than a complete "alternative medical system". It acts mainly by stimulating the nervous system, and its known modes of action include local antidromic axon reflexes, segmental and extrasegmental neuromodulation, and other central nervous system effects. Western medical acupuncture is principally used by conventional healthcare practitioners, most commonly in primary care. It is mainly used to treat musculoskeletal pain, including myofascial trigger point pain. It is also effective for postoperative pain and nausea. Practitioners of Western medical acupuncture tend to pay less attention than classical acupuncturists to choosing one point over another, though they generally choose classical points as the best places to stimulate the nervous system. The design and interpretation of clinical studies is constrained by lack of knowledge of the appropriate dosage of acupuncture, and the likelihood that any form of needling used as a usual control procedure in "placebo controlled" studies may be active. Western medical acupuncture justifies an unbiased evaluation of its role in a modern health service.

3. Local acupuncture style (局部针法)

In all of the following local acupuncture styles, the acupuncture points used are located on the local part of the body. These styles follow the Holographic theory. This means that one part of the body contains information for the whole body. Stimulating one spot can influence the function of a correlated part of the whole body.

(1) Auricular acupuncture style (耳针)

Auricular acupuncture style[106] stimulates points on the ear. The idea is that the ear contains information about the whole body. Each small spot on the ear is related to the function of a specific part of the whole body (e.g. the Holographic theory) (Figure 14). During treatment, the acupuncturist stimulates the exact co-related part of the ear to solve the disorder of the body. For example, for cervical spondylosis, the acupuncturist stimulates the spot for neck, elbow, and wrist points on the ear. But for inner organ diseases, a Western medicine concept is needed to decide the acupuncture points that need to be stimulated. For example for the coronary heart disease, we need to choose the heart point, but also have to stimulate the kidney point, sympathia point, endocrine point, adrenal gland point, and subcortical aphasia point on the ear.

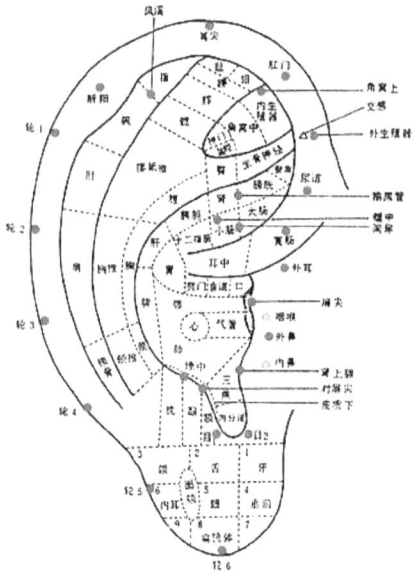

Figure 14. Acupuncture points on ear.[107]

The acupuncturist may also need TCM diagnosis to select proper points to stimulate. For example, for the treatment of conjunctivitis, the acupuncturist needs to stimulate not only the eye point, but also the liver point on the ear, because in TCM, the eye is associated with the Liver system in the body.

The points on the ear can be stimulated by various means, such as acupuncture needle, magnetic beards, imbedded needle, warm needle, electro-acupuncture, point injection, ion penetration, moxibustion, bleeding, etc.

(2) Scalp acupuncture (头皮针)

There are as many as ten kinds of scalp acupuncture styles.[108] In some, acupuncture points are selected based on the projection of brain functional zones on the scalp, some using the traditional acupuncture meridian system, or a combination. The scalp acupuncture introduced in most acupuncture textbooks is modified from the Jiao's scalp acupuncture style (see below).

(2.1) Jiao Sun-Fa Scalp acupuncture style (焦顺发头皮针)

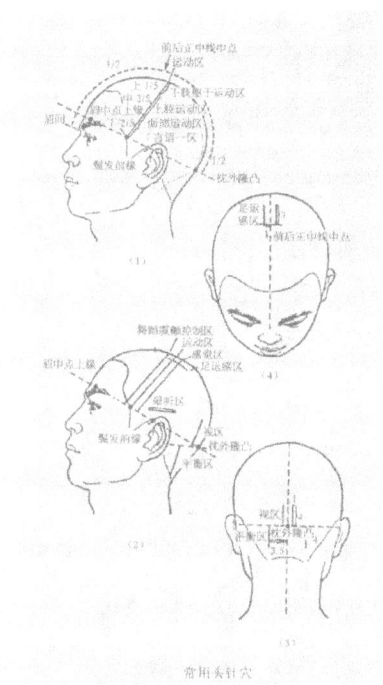

Figure 15. Acupuncture zones in scalp (Jiao's scalp acupuncture).[109]

This style was developed by Dr. Jiao Sun-Fa.[110] He believes that the functional regions of the brain are reflected and projected onto the scalp (Figure 15). Stimulating the corresponding area of the scalp can treat diseases that are associated with the functional region of the brain. The style is mostly used to treat brain-associated diseases. For example, to treat motor disorders, the acupuncturist can stimulate the motor region on the scalp. For the treatment of tremor paralysis and chorea, the acupuncturist stimulates the dance-tremor region. The functional regions of the brain are separated into the motor region, sensation region, dance-tremor region, dizziness-hearing region, feet motor-sensation region, vision region, and balance region.

(2.2) Fang Yun-Peng scalp acupuncture style (方云鹏头皮针)

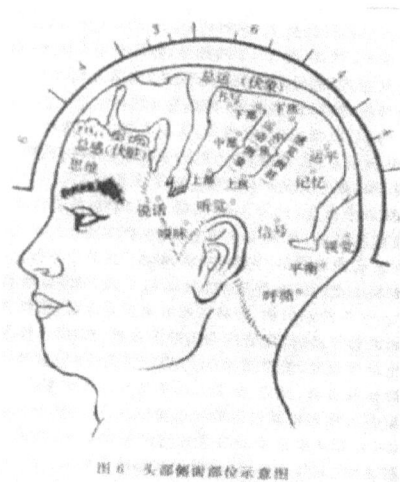

Figure 16. Acupuncture points on scalp (Fang's scalp acupuncture).[111]

This acupuncture style was founded by Dr. Fang Yun-Peng in the 1970s. It separates the surface of the scalp into four major regions (called Face-down diagram, Face-down organs, Reverse-diagram, Reverse organs) and eleven functional stimulation zones (for thinking, memory, speaking, motion, signal, hearing, vision, balance, breath and circulation) (Figure 16). It works much better for diseases in the nerve system (such as migraine, paralysis, and stroke) and also for rheumatic arthritis.

During the acupuncture treatment, the needle is inserted very quickly and vertically into the scalp and touches the bone membrane. This style of acupuncture emphasizes pulse diagnosis to decide which scalp regions to stimulate.

There is another scalp acupuncture style called Zhu Long-Yu scalp acupuncture. The distribution of the body on the scalp is similar to the Fang style, but it is opposite: the head region is on the rear of the scalp but the tail part is on the front. Both styles work well. This is not hard to understand, because in body acupuncture styles, the acupuncture points on the feet can be used to treat headache, suggesting that the head and the foot are correlated.

(2.3)   Zhu Ming-Qing scalp acupuncture style (朱明清头皮针)

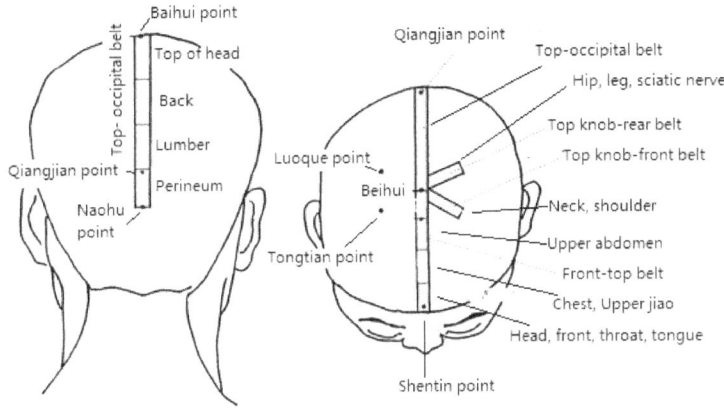

Figure 17. Acupuncture points on Scalp (Zhu's scalp acupuncture).[112]

This style was developed by Dr. Zhu Ming-Qing. He found that there are nine treatment belts on the scalp (Figure 17): Forehead-top belt, beside forehead I belt, beside forehead II belt, Top-temporal belt, Top-Occipital belt, Top-knob front belt, Top-knob rear belt, Front-temporal belt, Behind-temporal belt. Each belt is related to one part of the body. The acupuncture points chosen depend on the location of the sick part of the body. For example, for the treatment of sciatic pain, the acupuncturist stimulates the Top-knob front belt, because this belt is associated to the back part of the hip and the leg.

The following examples show the functions of each region on the scalp for acupuncture treatment:

The Forehead-top belt can be further separated into the first ¼, the second ¼, the third ¼ and the back ¼ part. The first ¼ part corresponds to diseases in the face, throat, and tongue. The second ¼ part corresponds to diseases in the chest (respiratory and heart). The third ¼ part corresponds to diseases in the upper abdomen (liver, gall bladder, stomach, spleen). The last ¼ part corresponds to diseases in the lower abdomen (kidney, urine bladder, prostate, uterus, ovary, anus).

The Beside forehead I belt corresponds to acute diseases in the middle Jiao (stomach, spleen, liver, gall bladder, pancreas).

The Beside forehead II belt corresponds to acute diseases in the lower Jiao (kidney, urine bladder, and reproductive system).

The Top-temporal belt is further separated into the upper 1/3 part, middle 1/3 part and lower 1/3 part. The upper 1/3 part corresponds to the diseases in lower limbs. The middle 1/3 part corresponds to the diseases in upper limb. The lower 1/3 part corresponds to the diseases in the face.

The Top-occipital belt, from the head top to the occipital, is for the diseases in the head, neck, back, lower back, and perineal part.

This is also a straight-forward scalp style that chooses acupuncture points on the scalp that correspond to the anatomic parts of the body. For example, for the treatment of lower back pain, the acupuncturist can stimulate the lower 1/3 part of the Top-occipital belt (back of head). During acupuncture, pulling-inserting technique is used.[32]

(2.4)   Liu Bing-Quan scalp acupuncture style (刘炳权八卦头针)

This is a style used by Dr. Liu Bing-Quan. Choose several acupuncture points on the scalp, then insert needles around the spot using the Eight-diagram (all the diagrams around) (Figure 18). The distance from the edge needles to the center of the Eight- diagram is different; there is both a small and bigger Eight-diagram in the scalp. This is similar to the Around Acupuncture technique. For the treatment, we may need only one Eight-diagram acupuncture (big or small Eight-diagram), or use two or three Eight-diagram circles on the scalp. Apparently it is not a typical Eight-diagram as we use it in other part of the body. For example, when the Eight-diagram is used on the abdomen, the spots on the diagram have to take into consideration their related meaning to the disease we are treating.

---

[32] Most scalp acupuncture styles use twist technique, not the pulling-inserting technique.

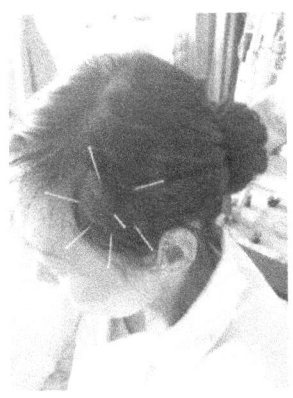

Figure 18. Head Eight-diagram acupuncture.[113]

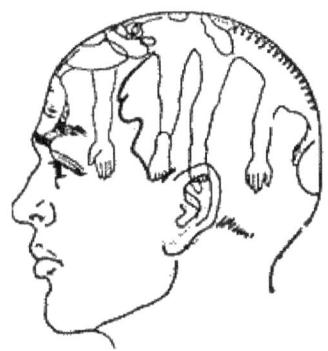

Figure 19. Acupuncture point distribution in Tang's scalp acupuncture style.

(2.5)   Tang Song-Yan scalp acupuncture style (汤颂延头针)

This scalp acupuncture was developed by Dr. Tang Song-Yan.[114] He found that the projection of body parts on the scalp is as in Figure 19. Stimulation on that part on the scalp can treat the disease on the corresponding part of the body.

(2.6)   Lin Xue-Jian scalp acupuncture style (林学俭头针刺激新区)

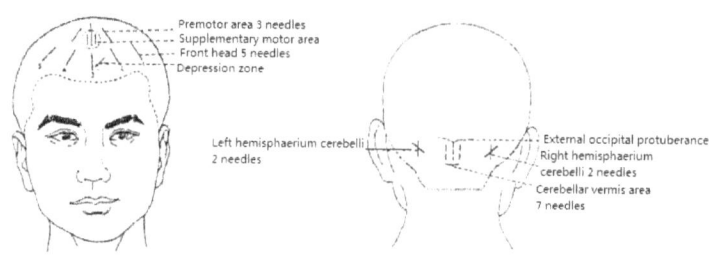

Figure 20. Acupuncture point distribution in Lin's scalp acupuncture style.**Error! Bookmark not defined.**

This scalp acupuncture style was developed by Dr. Lin Xue-Jian.[115] It works on several regions on the scalp (Figure 20): Temporal-three-needle region; Fronthead-five-needle region; Front-motor region; Attached-motor region; Depression region; Small-brain region (two needles on left side and tow on right side); and Small-brain-seven-needle region (on rear of head).

(2.7)   Yu Chang-De scalp acupuncture style (俞昌德头针)

This scalp acupuncture style was developed by Dr. Yu Chang-De.[116] The acupuncture needles are inserted mostly along the skull gap.

(2.8)   Jin Rui scalp acupuncture style (靳瑞头针)

This scalp acupuncture style was developed by Dr. Jin Rui (靳瑞 1932-2010).[117] Similar to his three-needle group of acupuncture on other parts of body, he also uses three needles as a group on the scalp for treatment. The acupuncture points are the traditional acupuncture points for the scalp. For example, for the treatment of poor intelligence, the needles used are the following: two needles on the Benshen acupuncture points (one on left and another on the right side). This three-needle group is called intelligence three-needle. For the treatment of a motor disorder, and poor balance, the three needles used are the Naohu and the Naoshi (one on the left and another on the right). It is called Brain-three-needle acupuncture.

(2.9)   Toshikatsu scalp acupuncture style (山元敏胜新头针)

This scalp acupuncture style was developed by Japanese acupuncturist Toshikatsu Yamamoto.[118] He uses acupuncture on several lines in the front of the head (Figure 21). Most of the acupuncture points are on the edge of the hair. There are points A, B, C, D, and E.

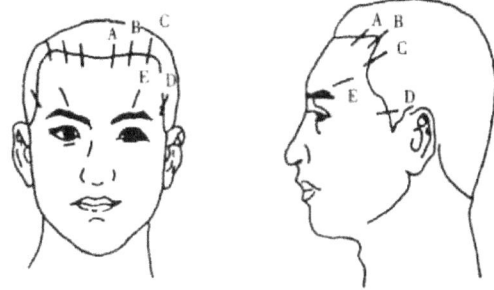

Figure 21. Acupuncture point distribution in Toshikatsu's scalp acupuncture style.[118]

Point A: for the treatment of spondylosis, stiff neck, rear headache.
Point B: for the treatment of shoulder pain.
Point C: for shoulder and upper limb.
Point D: for lower back and lower limb.
Point E: for problems in the chest.

(3) Face acupuncture style (面针)

There two types of facial acupuncture styles, traditional facial acupuncture and new facial acupuncture style. The major difference between them is the distribution of acupuncture points on the face. For traditional style, the acupuncture points are distributed across whole face, while in the new style, the points are distributed mostly in the middle part of the face.

(3.1)   Traditional facial acupuncture (传统面针)

Facial acupuncture style separates the face into seven regions (Figure 22).[119] They are front head region, nose region, eye region, mouth region, ear region, cheek region and cheekbone region.

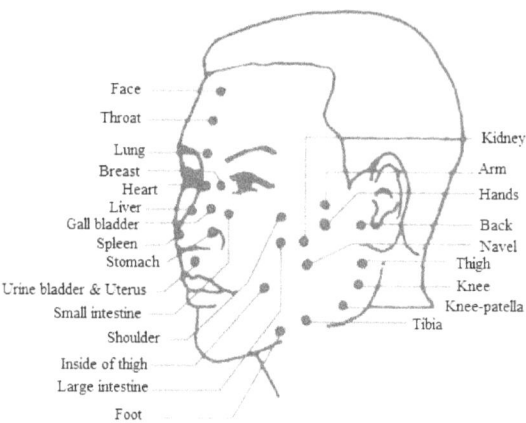

Figure 22. Acupuncture point distribution in traditional facial acupuncture style[119]

There are two ways to select acupuncture points. Firstly, the points can be chosen as the corresponding acupuncture point on the face for the body part. For example, if there is stomach pain, the acupuncturist can stimulate the stomach point on the face. Secondly, we can choose based on TCM diagnosis. For example for the treatment of insomnia, if it is diagnosed as a Liver and Kidney Yin deficiency, the acupuncturist stimulates the liver point and the kidney point.

The facial points are mostly used to stop pain, however, they are also used for acupuncture anesthesia. For example, for total gastric resection, the acupuncturist stimulates the stomach, lung, heart and spleen points on the face. Facial acupuncture also works for the treatment of neurosis, hypertension, arthritis, and asthma.

Facial acupuncture must induce the Deqi sensation.

(3.2)   New facial acupuncture (新面针)

New facial acupuncture was introduced by Dr. Huang Ying-Li.[120] The acupuncture points are selected with the corresponding relationship between the name of the points on the face and the name of the body part (Figure 23). The acupuncture points can also be decided according to TCM diagnosis (as with traditional facial acupuncture).

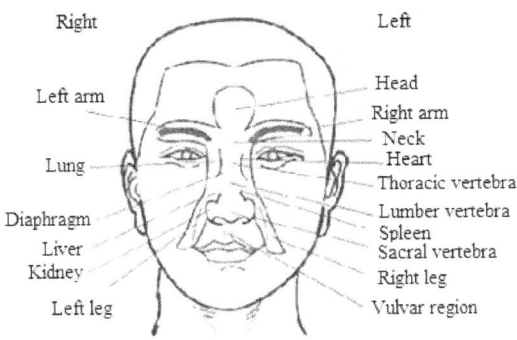

Figure 23. Acupuncture point distribution in traditional facial acupuncture style. [120]

Clinical experience shows that new facial acupuncture works both for painful syndromes and for post-stroke syndromes.

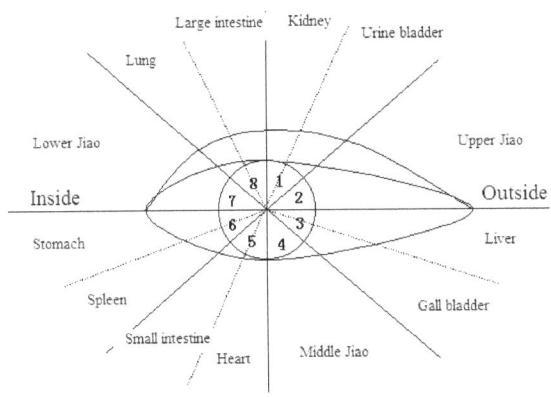

Figure 24. Acupuncture zones in left eye. [121]

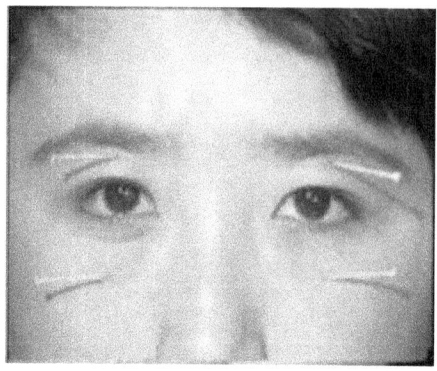

Figure 25. Eye acupuncture. [122]

(4) Peng Jin-Shan Eye acupuncture style (彭静山眼针疗法)

Eye acupuncture style was originally founded by Dr. Peng Jin-Shan, and later further developed by Dr. Tian Wei-Zhu. [123]

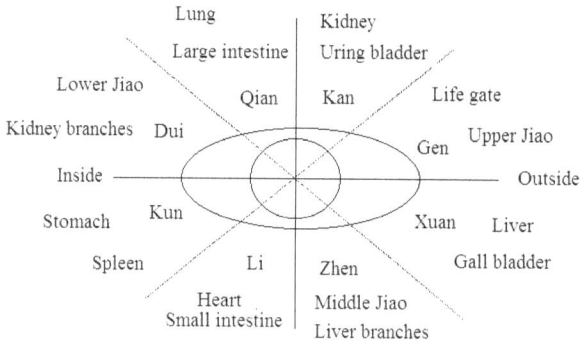

Figure 26. Eight-diagram distribution in eye (left).[124]

Each eye is separated into various regions (Figure 24, 25). There are several ways to choose acupuncture points around the eye. First, choose the point according to the meridian. If the pain is in the Lung meridian, stimulate the point on the Lung point on the eye. Second, choose it according to the local branch blood vessel, by seeing which region has more red-colored blood vesicles. Lastly, choose according to which Jiao cavity the disease is in. If the disease is in the upper Jiao cavity (inside the chest), stimulate the Upper Jiao point on the eye. If it is in the Middle Jiao, such as with stomach pain, stimulate the Middle Jiao on the eye. The points can also be chosen according to Eight-diagram in the eyes (Figure 26).

The problem with eye acupuncture is that it is easy to cause bleeding. To prevent this, it is recommended to use thin and short needles and to use an ice-cold compress on the eye before acupuncture. Sensation of Deqi is required.

It is summarized that eye acupuncture is good for both the treatment of pain syndromes and post-stroke syndromes too.

(5) Nose acupuncture style (鼻针)

For this acupuncture style,[125] the acupuncture points are on the nose in three lines, with 23 stimulation points. (Figure 27) The principle in the selection of acupuncture points on the nose for the treatment is the same as for facial acupuncture.

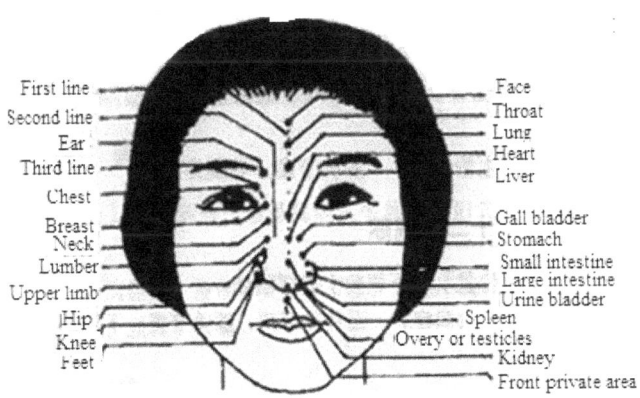

Figure 27. Acupuncture point distribution on nose.[126]

The sensitive spot on the nose can be found by pressing with a probe on the nose, or by electric detecting tip. This works better to stimulate the sensitive spot.

Nose acupuncture is used for acupuncture anesthesia. The basic points are the ear and lung points. Depending on the part of the surgery, other points are also used in combination.

(6) Tongue acupuncture style (舌针)

There are acupuncture points on the top of the tongue and beneath it too (Figure 28).[127] The TCM diagnosis, in consideration of the color, the shape, the wet or dryness, and the flexibility, of the tongue, is needed in selection of acupuncture points for the treatment.

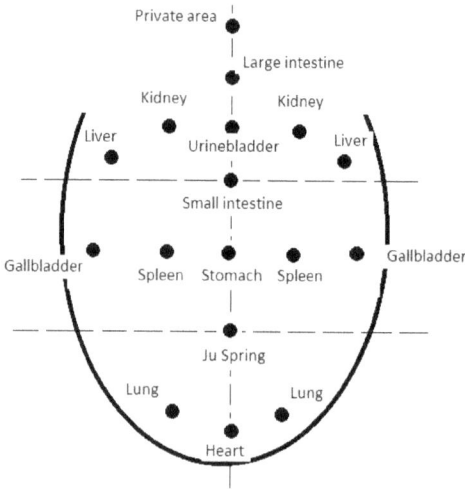

Figure 28. Acupuncture point distribution on tongue. [127]

For example, for the treatment of poor sleep, the heart point, the kidney point and the front head point are chosen from the tongue for the acupuncture. Because there are no points corresponding to the limbs, shoulder or back, to treat diseases in the muscle and joint pains in these areas of the body, acupuncture points outside of the tongue must also be used.

The acupuncture points on the tongue may be pierced with acupuncture needles, or pouched for bleeding therapy. With needle acupuncture, the Deqi sensation is needed, with the twist technique or the pulling-inserting technique.

Tongue acupuncture is mostly used for the treatment of tongue-related diseases, or body motor disorders, such as tongue numbness, tongue skew, tongue stiffness, ulcer in tongue, bad smell from mouth, post-stroke syndrome, and paralysis, though it is also used for the treatment of disorders in the circulation system, hypertension and spondylosis.

(7) Mouth acupuncture style (口针)

Mouth acupuncture was developed by Dr. Liu Jin-Rong.[128] The acupuncture points are distributed on the mucus of mouth, under the tongue (Figure 29).

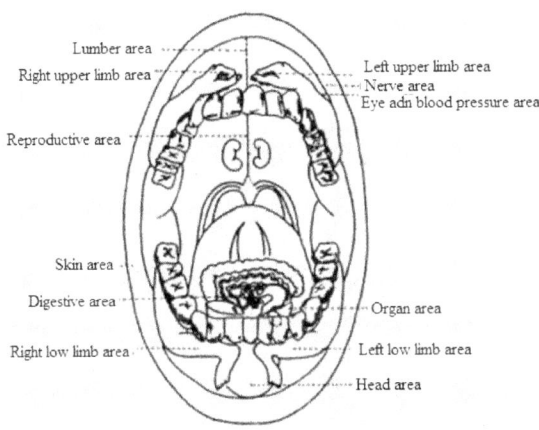

Figure 29. Acupuncture point distribution on mouth.[128]

The acupuncture points on the mouth are selected for treatment in a similar way as for facial acupuncture and nose acupuncture. For example, for the treatment of sciatic pain, the sciatic point plus the hip point are selected for stimulation. The points are cross selected. For example, if the pain is in left side of the body, the right point in the mouth is selected.

This acupuncture requires the Deqi sensation. It works better for various pain syndromes, such as sciatic pain and acute strain on the lower back. It also works well for paralysis.[129]

(8) Ren-zhong acupuncture style (人中针)

This acupuncture style aims to stimulate acupuncture points on the Ren-zhong groove (e.g. the nasolabial groove).[130] There are nine acupuncture points in the groove. From the mouth lip up to the nose are points 1 to 9, all of which can work for diseases in the face and head. Also, points 1 to 3 can work for diseases in the Upper Jiao part of the body. Points 4 to 6 are for the Middle Jiao of the body and points 7 to 9 are for the Lower Jiao part of the body.

If the needle tip tilts to the left side, treatment works better for the diseases on the left side of the body. Similarly, if the tip leans towards the right, it works more for the diseases on the right side of the body. If it leans towards the head, it works for the diseases along the Du meridian, such as in the face, head, neck, and back. If it leans towards the stomach, it works more for diseases along the Ren meridian, such as with chest pain or stomach pain.

Usually only one needle is used on the groove. If needed, treatment would be combined with body acupuncture, unless it is used for a stroke, for which more needles may be used in the groove.

(9) Foot acupuncture style (足针)

Besides the acupuncture points that belong to traditional acupuncture style, there are different acupuncture styles in the foot (Figure 30). [131,132]

The acupuncture points for this style are selected for treatment in a similar way as for palm acupuncture, nose acupuncture, etc. For example, for the treatment of a headache, the acupuncturist can stimulate the head point on the foot. For the treatment of stomach pain, the acupuncturist uses acupuncture on the stomach point on the foot.

The point chosen can also be selected according to TCM diagnosis. For example, for the treatment of dizziness, if it is diagnosed as Liver-kidney Yin deficiency, the acupuncturist needs to use acupuncture on the head point, and the liver and kidney points as well. The Deqi sensation is required.

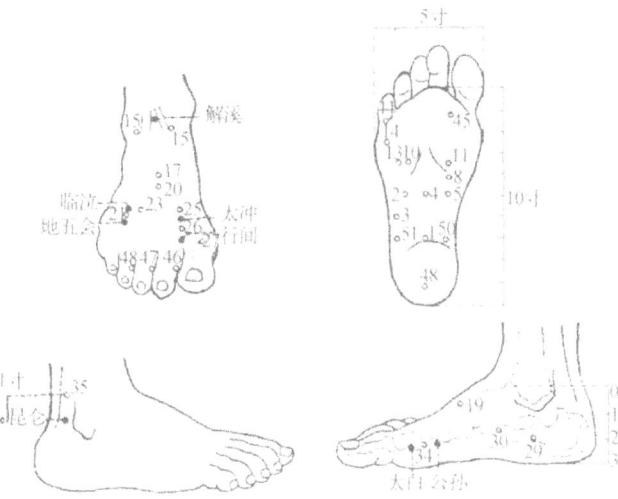

Figure 30. Acupuncture point on Foot acupuncture style (round and the numbered dot). Red dots mean the acupuncture points belong to traditional acupuncture style.

(10)   Fang Ben-Zheng Foot region acupuncture style (足象针)

Foot region acupuncture and Hand region acupuncture (see below) were developed by Dr. Fang Ben-Zheng.[133] Similar to ear acupuncture, the acupuncture points in the feet can also be distributed roughly as a human being figure (Figure 31).

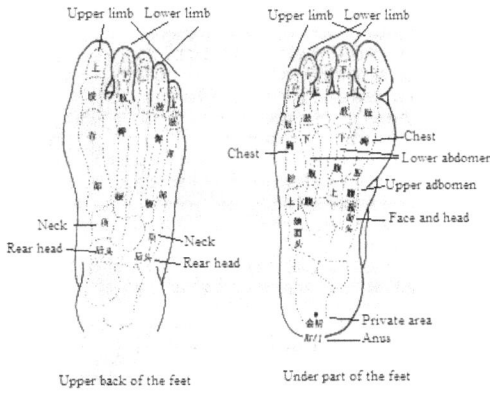

Figure 31. Foot diagram picture. [134]

(11)   Hand acupuncture (手针针法)

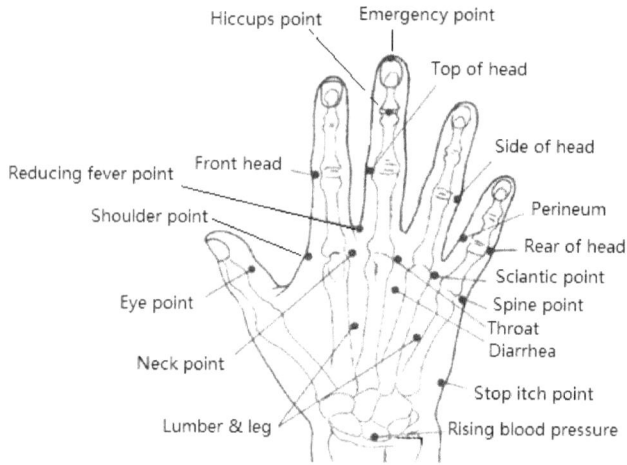

Figure 32. Acupuncture points on back of hand.[135]

There is also an acupuncture style for hands (Figure. 32, 33).[136] Stimulation of the acupuncture points on the hands works for the treatment of various diseases.

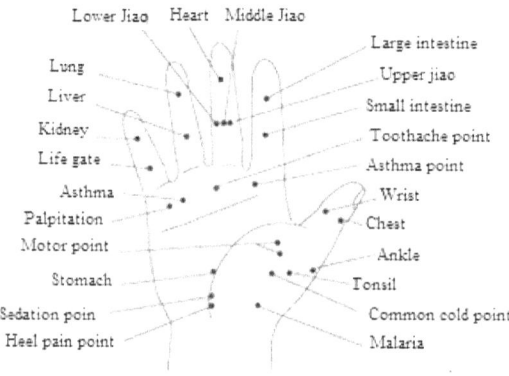

Figure 33. Acupuncture points on palm side of hand.[135]

(12)   Hand region acupuncture style (手象针针法)

There is different distribution pattern for acupuncture points on hands. This is called Hand region acupuncture (Figure 34). **Error! Bookmark not defined.**

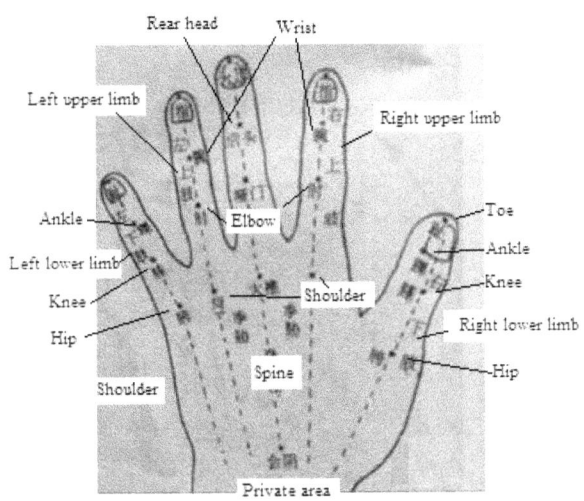

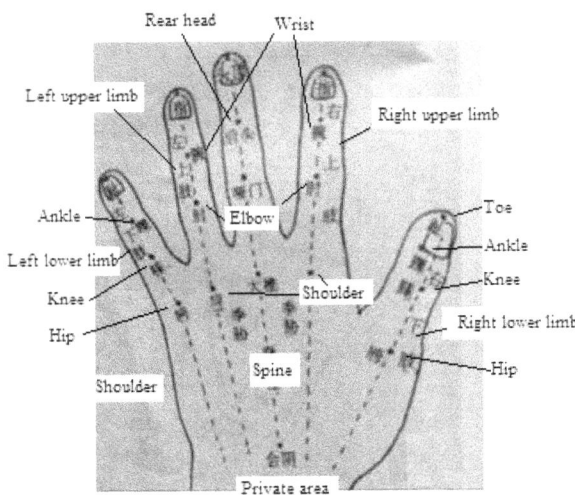

Figure 34. Acupuncture points and zones in hand (both sides). [134]

(13)   Yu Hao Yin-Yang Nine-acupuncture style (余浩阴阳九针)

This style was developed by Dr. Yu Hao.[137, 138] The needles are mostly applied on fingers (For male, use left hand, for female, use right hand). The primary theory of this style is that a hand contains information for the whole body, as does a finger (Figure 35, 36, 37).

There are basically nine kinds of acupuncture techniques used with this style of acupuncture. Pulse diagnosis is used to facilitate diagnosis and the decision of which acupuncture technique to use.

For example, if a patient suffers from a stiff neck, the acupuncturist can use acupuncture on the spot on the thumb where it represents the neck (the second thumb finger joints). The needle can be in either direction, either from the thumb tip to the thumb root, or from the root to its tip (Figure 38).

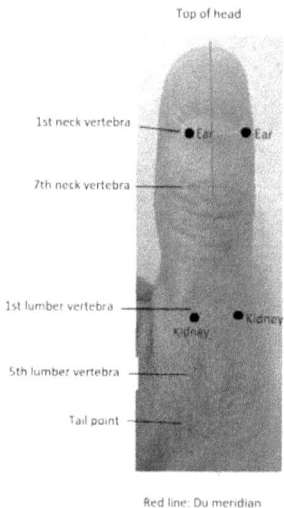

Figure 35. Acupuncture zones on back of thumb in Yu's acupuncture style (modified).[137]

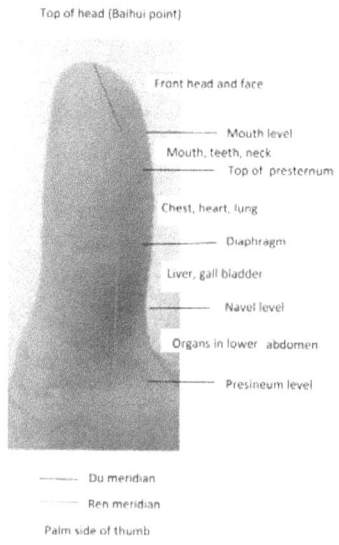

Figure 36. Acupuncture zones on palm side of thumb in Yu's acupuncture style (modified).[137]

(14)   Ma Chun-Hui Small Six-He acupuncture (马春晖小六合针法)

This acupuncture style was created by Dr. Ge Qin-Fu (葛钦甫) [139] and developed by Dr. Ma Chun-Hui. It also works in palm. [140, 141] The acupuncture point is selected according to the Eight-diagram theory on the palm (Figure 39,40). It usually uses only one needle and is called One-needle acupuncture technique.

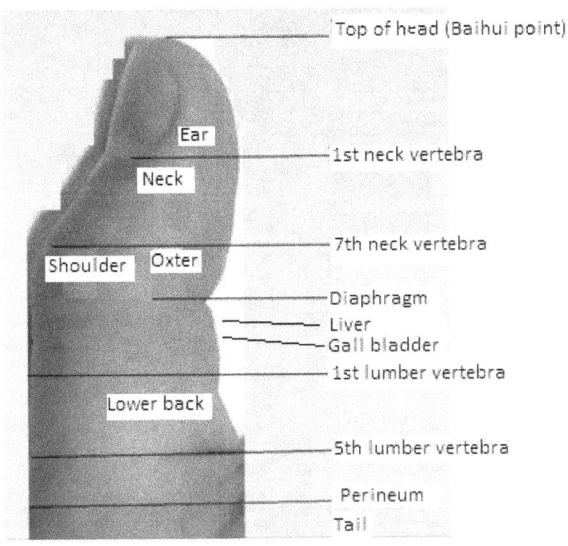

Figure 37. Acupuncture zones on side of thumb in Yu's acupuncture style (modified).[137]

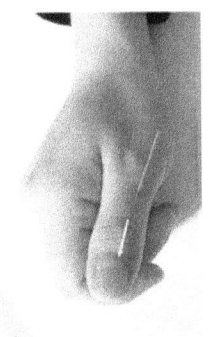

Figure 38. Acupuncture zones on side of thumb in Yu's acupuncture style (modified).[137]

It does not require the Deqi sensation. There is almost no pain.

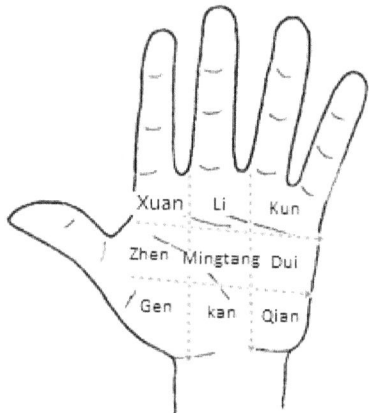

Figure 39. Distribution pattern of palm Eight-diagram.[142]

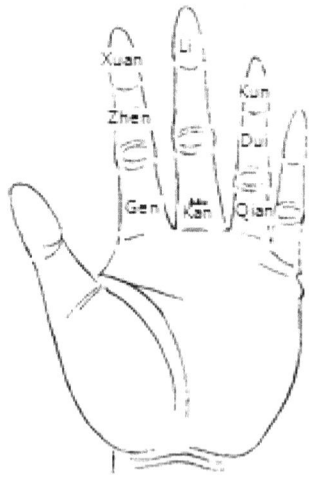

Figure 40. Finger Eight-diagram pattern.[143]

(15)   Ge Qin-Fu Taiji Si-He acupuncture style (葛钦甫腹部太极六合针法)

This style was developed by Dr. Ge Qin-Fu. **Error! Bookmark not defined.** This style of acupuncture uses the Eight-diagram theory in the abdomen. There are three levels of the Eight-diagram diagrams (Figure 41). Two Eight-diagram diagrams are in the abdomen and the third expands to the whole body. In the abdomen, the diagrams are called Inner Eight-diagram diagram, and Middle Eight-diagram diagram, both are centered with the navel. The Inner Eight-diagram is a square with1.5 body cun from the center of the navel, and the Middle Eight-diagram is also a square of 4 body cun from the center of the navel.

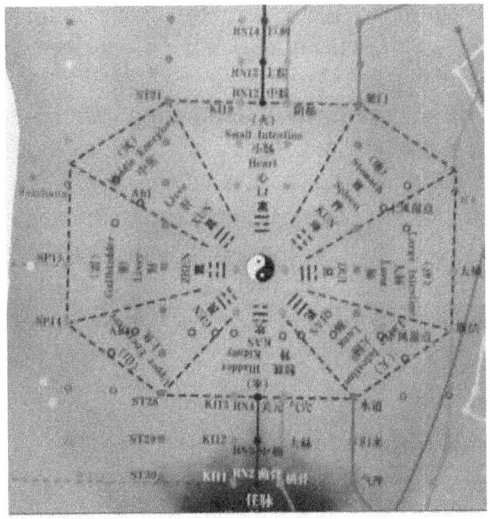

Figure 41. Distribution of abdominal Eight-diagram around the navel.[144]

For treatment, the acupuncture points are chosen depending on the relationship and association of the diagram zone and the body parts (the head, neck, limbs), as well as the function of the body parts. For example, if a patient has pain on the right arm, the acupuncturist can insert a needle in the Zhen and Xun diagrams. This is because the two diagrams mimic the direction of the right upper part of the body (the right arm). This is also because the diagram is associated with body tendon and nerve. Both diagrams maintain the normal function of the tendon and nervous system. If a patient has a mouth ulcer, the acupuncturist can chose to do acupuncture on the Dui diagram, because the Dui diagram is responding to the normal function of mouth.

Acupuncture points are selected based on several theories. For example, they can be selected simply with the space/geographic correlation of the diagram and the body part (as above) or as functional correlation of the diagram and the meridians. For example, if the sick meridian is detected as Hand Yin meridian, the acupuncturist can select the Gen and the Zhen diagrams, because these two diagrams are associated with the Yin meridian. The acupuncture points can also be selected as a time circle of Zi Yu Liu Zhu theory, the Five-element theory, etc.

Having chosen the diagram(s), insert needles into the diagram (the exact point is not so important, but should be within the diagram/zone), with needle tips pointing towards the edge of the body (away from the middle vertical line of the body). Deqi sensation is not emphasized. The patient does not feel very much pain. The needle can be left in place for about 30 min. The needle in the Inner Eight-diagram is needed. To enhance the healing effect, another needle is inserted into the Middle diagram but in the same diagram as in the Inner Diagram (It is called a directive needle. One needle is enough). Sometimes, acupuncturist even use more needles on the Outer Eight-diagram (accepting needle), or in the sick part or sick meridian (enhancing needle), to enhance the healing effect. This is called the four-step acupuncture program (四部通调).

(16)   Dr. Bo Zhi-Yun Abdominal acupuncture style (薄智云腹针疗法)

This abdominal acupuncture was developed by Dr. Bo Zhi-Yun.[145]

In this style, acupuncture points are, most of the time, the same as in traditional meridians, but the needle is inserted very shallowly (Figure 42). The patient does not feel any typical Deqi sensation.

This style of acupuncture needs very precise location of acupuncture points on the abdomen and precise sequence of needle insertion and removal. The needles are manipulated only with twist (not pulling up and down), or with slight twist and very slow pulling up and down. To remove the needle, the needles that were inserted first will be removed first (do not insert them deeper before removing).

For example, in the treatment of a stiff neck, the acupuncture points used are Zhongwan, Shangqu and Huaroumen, all of which belong to the traditional meridian system. It is necessary to insert the needle into Zhongwan first, then Shangqu, followed by Huaroumen last. The needle on Zhongwan needs to be inserted deeply, Shangqu shallowly, and Huaroumen at middle depth.[146]

Needle retention time is usually 20-30 min. It can be a longer time for chronic disease or if the body constitution is stronger. Acupuncture should be performed once a day for three days, then changed to once every other day. Six to ten sessions are one healing course.

It should be mentioned that the measurement of the distance on the abdomen in this style of acupuncture is unusual: it is the project distance, not the actual skin surface distance (Figure 43).

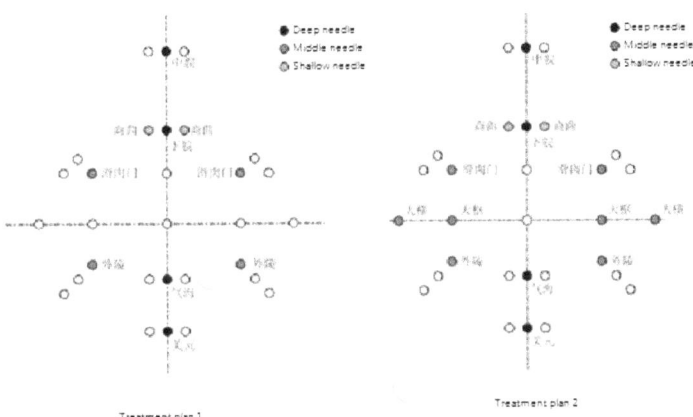

Figure 42. Example of acupuncture points used in Bo's abdominal acupuncture style, with deep, middle deep or shallow acupuncture insertion.[147]

Generally speaking, Abdomen acupuncture is used for inner-oriented diseases, chronic diseases, or complex diseases. It is not recommended for acute abdominal syndrome, varicomphaius, neoplasm metastasis in abdomen, pregnancy for more than 3 months, or if the patient is very weak in body condition.

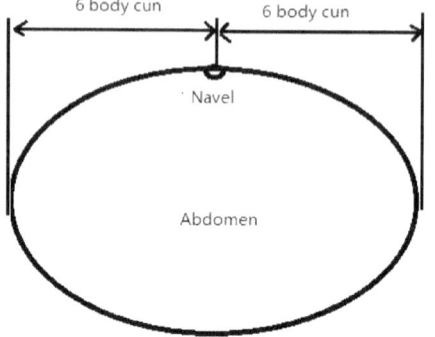

6 body cun   6 body cun

Navel

Abdomen

Measurement of distance from navel to side of abdomen:
project distance, not actual distance on skin

Figure 43. Illustration of the way to measure distance on abdomen in the Bo's acupuncture style.

One of the special characteristics of Abdomen acupuncture is that there is fixed acupuncture formula for each disease. For example, the location and the number of acupuncture points, and the depth of the needle in each point, are all standardized. These requirements have to be followed exactly.

(17)   Sun Shen-Tian Abdominal Acupuncture style (孙申田腹针疗法)

Sun's abdominal acupuncture style was developed by Dr. Sun Shen-Tian.[148] It separates the abdomen into ten zones (Figure 44). Zones 1-4 are located in the upper abdomen; zones 5-7 are in the lower abdomen; zones 8 and 9 are around the navel; and zone 10 is on the anterior superior iliac spine.

The zones are separated as follows: along the middle vertical line from metasternum to navel, four horizontally zones are separated equally. Zone 1 is on the top next to the metasternum. Zone 2 follows, then zone 3, and zone 4 is next to the navel. Similarly, the area from the navel to the synchondroses pubis, is also equally separated into 3 horizontal zones. Zone 5 is next to the navel, zone 7 is next to the synchondroses pubis, and zone 6 is in between zones 5 and 7. In zone 1, there are 3 acupuncture points. In zones 2 to 7, each zone has two points (0.5 body cun to the middle vertical line of abdomen, middle to the upper and lower board of next zones, one point on each side of the abdominal middle line). In zone 8, there are 4 points. They are 0.5 body cun around the navel: left, right, top and bottom of the navel. Zone 9 is 0.5 body cun above the navel, then 1 body cun to the left and right, then from this point draw a vertical line 2 cm long. For zone 10, from the anterior superior iliac spine, draw a vertical line (parallel to the middle line of the abdomen).

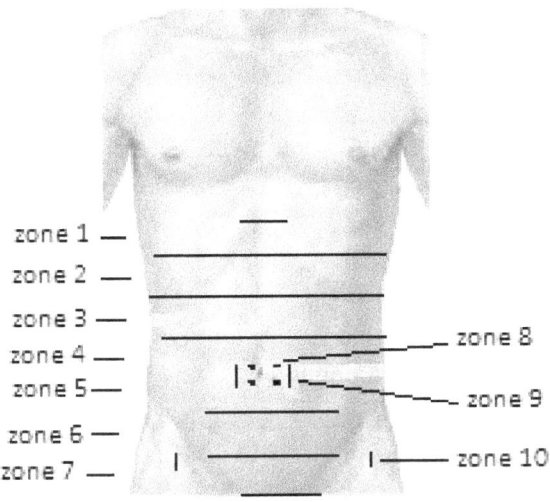

Figure 44. Acupuncture zones in Sun's Abdominal Acupuncture style.

Zone 1: There three acupuncture points in this zone. This is the emotional zone. It works for anxiety, depression, cravings, poor sleep, heavy dreams, poor memory.

Zone 2: This zone is for adjustment of autonomic nerve and endocrine functions (2 points, left and right side). It works for primary hypertension, diabetes, menopause syndrome, etc.

Zone 3: This zone is for vocal paralysis. It works for Parkinson's disease, tourettes syndrome, chorea.

Zone 4: This is the motion zone. It works for disorders of motor functions and post-stroke syndrome.

Zone 5: This zone is under the navel, and is the sensation zone. It works for various disorders in body sensation, such as pain and numbness.

Zone 6: This is also a motion Zone. It works for paralysis.

Zone 7: This is the vision zone. It works for disorders in vision.

Zone 8: The functions here are similar to zone 1.

Zone 9: This is the Foot Sensation-Motion zone. It works for restless leg, lower limb pain, urinary diseases, and diseases in perineal position area.

Zone 10: This is the Balance zone. It works for disorders of balance due to a small brain.

For most acupuncture points, the needles are inserted obliquely, except for needles in zone 8, in which the needles can be inserted vertically. Deqi sensation is required.

Sun's abdominal acupuncture is a newly developed acupuncture style. Currently, it is used in combination with other acupuncture styles.[149, 150]

(18)   Qi Yong Navel acupuncture (齐永脐针)

Navel acupuncture style was developed by Dr. Qi Yong.[151] There are several ways to select acupuncture points in the navel acupuncture style (Figure 45).[152] Points can be selected by locating a pain spot under pressure, by finding a knob under the skin, by using Luoshu Holographic distribution, by using Eight-zone Holographic distribution, by using Five-element distribution, and by using Earth-branch Holographic distribution.

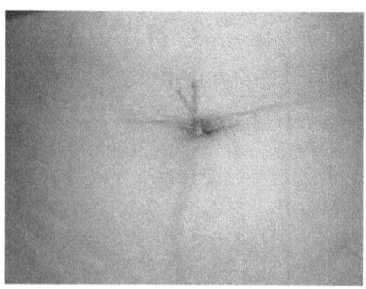

Figure 45. Navel acupuncture.[152]

(a). Painful spot navel acupuncture

Find the painful spot around the wall of the navel. Stimulate the painful spot with a needle for several minutes. The tip of the needle points towards the wall (not vertically towards the bottom of the abdomen). About 20% of patients can have such painful spots. It is easier to find the painful spot with acute diseases.

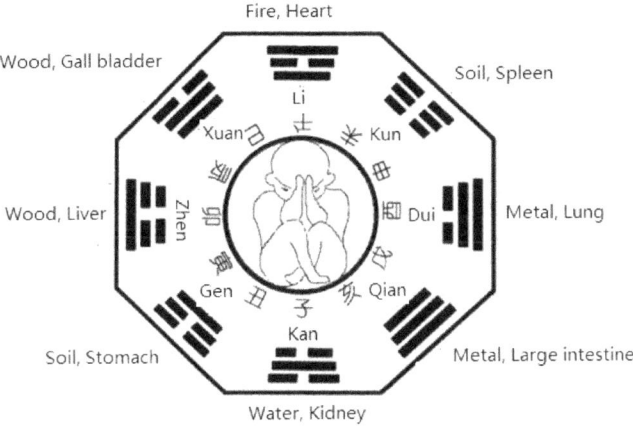

Figure 46. Diagram in Luo Shu style. The small figure in the center represents the direction of the body to each diagram.

(b). Knob navel acupuncture
Find a subcutaneous knob. The patient could feel pain upon pressing that spot. The skin color should be normal and the size of the knob should be about the same as a grain of rice. We only need to press the knob several times a day. Such subcutaneous knobs can be found in many patients with chronic diseases.

(c). Navel Luoshu Holographic acupuncture (洛书全息)

The navel contains information for the whole body. Distribution of the information in the navel is as follows (Figure 46):

Look at the small human being figure inside the picture. It represents the correlation of the direction of navel wall to the body. For example, the top wall of navel is related to the head, the bottom to the feet, the left side wall to the left arm (upper left) and left leg (lower left). If there is pain in the left shoulder, the acupuncturist stimulates the upper left wall of navel. If the pain is in the right hip, the acupuncturist stimulates the lower right wall of the navel. This style of acupuncture is often used for the treatment of muscle-joint disorders.

(d). Navel Eight-diagram navel acupuncture (后天八卦脐针)
The distribution of organs is based on the Eight-diagram picture (Figure 47). For example, in the treatment of respiratory diseases, the acupuncturist uses a needle to stimulate the left wall of the navel (left means the direction of left hand of the patient, though the spot is on the right of the following picture). For liver disease, the acupuncturist stimulates the right wall of the navel of patient.

(e). Five-element navel acupuncture (五行脐针疗法)
Make TCM diagnosis first, then perform acupuncture treatment, following the principle of the Five-element theory (following the Figure 46, above).

Using Co-relation theory of the Organ relationship (脏腑关系).
This means to directly stimulate the corresponding position on the navel wall, which has the same nature as the TCM diagnosed disease. For example for a liver disease, which belongs to Liver Wood in TCM, the acupuncturist stimulates the navel wall on the right side of the patient's trunk (it is the Zhen diagram, which belongs to Liver Wood). The acupuncturist can either stimulate the Gall bladder Xun position on the navel wall, which belongs to the Gall bladder position, because the Gall bladder and the Liver have a surface-inner relationship. In this example, it is called gross co-relation (大比合) to stimulate the diagram of the diseased diagram, and it is called small co-relation, (小比合) for the stimulation of another diagram, which has a surface-inner relationship with the diseased diagram.

Using mother-son theory of the Five-element theory (五行生克关系). If the disease belongs to weakness, perform acupuncture on its month diagram (previous meridian) position on the navel; and if the disease belongs to overwhelming condition, the acupuncturist stimulates the son diagram (following diagram). The acupuncture can also be performed in another way: for the overwhelming condition in a diagram, for example, Lung Fire, the acupuncturist can stimulate the Heart Fire diagram (with the needle tip pointing towards the head of the patient), because Heart Fire counteracts the Lung Metal. If the condition belongs to weakness, for example, Lung Weakness condition, the acupuncturist can stimulate the navel wall of the left hand direction of the patient (the Kun diagram/position/direction, which belongs to Spleen

Soil), since Spleen Soil nourishes Lung Metal. Similarly, the acupuncturist can also stimulate the middle bottom, the navel wall on the right leg direction of the patient (both belong to Soil).

If the needle is inserted vertically from the middle of the navel, it is balanced nourish-depletion technique and it is used to treat diseases of the digestive system (TCM spleen and stomach). If the needle is placed a little bit towards the up direction (the head direction), it is used for the treatment of heart disease and eye disease. If it is placed towards the foot direction (the Water and the Kidney direction), it is used for the treatment of diseases in the urinary system. If it is placed towards the right direction (the direction of the right hand of the patient, the Wood, the Liver direction), it is used for the treatment of liver disease. One needle and one spot can treat many kind of disease.

(f). Earth-branch of Eight-diagram based time navel acupuncture (地支八卦脐针)

Earth-branch Holographic acupuncture system (Figure 47) was developed by Dr. Guo Chang-Dian and Chen Wen (郭常典和陳文). It is mostly used for those diseases that show a very clear time-related onset pattern.[153, 154] This means that the disease recurs at a fixed time of the day, month or year.

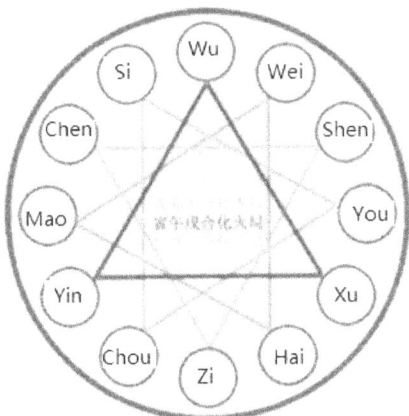

Figure 47. Earth-branch time circulation chart.[155]

According to the Chinese bio-clock, the bottom of the clock is midnight, the right side is 6 am, the top is 12 pm, and the left is 6 pm. For example, if the diarrhea happens always at 3 am, the acupuncturist can use a needle to stimulate the 7 pm position of the navel. The needle should be inserted horizontally or obliquely, but not vertically. If a cough always occurs at 5 pm, which is the 酉 time zone of Chinese clock and it located on the 3 pm of the ordinary clock, the acupuncturist can stimulate the 3 pm position of the navel wall. To stimulate the time-matched position, use the nourish-depletion technique of acupuncture.

For weak diseases, it is necessary to use nourishing technique by stimulating the next time zone on the navel wall. For the same cough patient, the acupuncturist needs to stimulate the navel wall of the patient in the 4 pm position. For overwhelming disease condition, the acupuncturist needs to use a depleting technique by stimulate the previous time zone. In the same cough example, the acupuncturist needs to insert the needle on his navel wall in the 2 pm position. This is position nourish-depletion technique.

The acupuncturist can also use handle technique for the nourish-depletion: strong stimulation belongs to depletion; keeping the needle in place for a while (retention) is nourishing. The position of nourish-depletion and the manual nourish-depletion technique can be combined at the same time.

(g). Four-diagram Navel acupuncture (四局针法) [156]

In Figure 47 above, if the acupuncturist uses three needles together in the combination pattern shown, the procedure can create different healing effects. For example, if the acupuncturist stimulates the navel wall on the Shen (Urine bladder), Zi (Gall bladder) and Chen (Stomach) position, it is called Water diagram (the yellow lines), which is used for the treatment of diseases that belong to Foot Yangming Stomach, Foot Shaoyang Gall bladder, and Foot Taiyang Urine bladder meridians.

If the acupuncturist stimulates the Ji (Spleen), You (Kidney) and Chou (Liver) (the blue lines), the procedure creates a Metal diagram, which is used for the treatment of diseases that are distributed in the range of the Foot Taiyin Spleen, Foot Shaoyin Kidney and Foot Jueyin Liver meridians.

If the acupuncturist stimulates the He (Three Jiao), Mao (Large intestine) and Wei (Small intestine) positions on the wall of navel (the green lines), this is the Wood diagram, which is used for the treatment of diseases that are distributed in the range of the Hand Taiyang Small intestine, Hand Shaoyang Three Jiao and Hand Yangming Large intestine meridians.

If the acupuncturist stimulates the Yin (Lung), Wu (Heart) and Shu (Heart shell) positions on the navel wall, the procedure creates a Fire diagram, which is used for the treatment of diseases that are distributed in the range of Hand Taiyin Lung, Shaoyin Heart and Jueyin Heart shell meridians.

Among these local acupuncture systems, the Auricular acupuncture, Scalp acupuncture, and the Abdomen acupuncture system are used more often. The Foot acupuncture system has been developed and used more in Western countries as reflexology.

The specific difference with the Abdomen acupuncture style is that it requires no feeling from the acupuncture needle by patients (similar to the Floating acupuncture and Wrist-ankle acupuncture systems above)

(19)   Holographic acupuncture system (全息针灸体系)

Holographic acupuncture system was created by Dr. Zhang Ying-Qing.[157] The main idea of the theory is that any small part of the body contains information for the whole body (Figure 48, 49, 50). Indeed it has been found that many small parts of the body can be stimulated to treat diseases in other parts of the body. The distribution of the points in the small part of the body can cover the anatomic structure of the whole body. The smallest part of the body is found to be as simple as a single bone (Figure 29). The Holographic theory is frequently used to explain the function of some acupuncture points in the treatment.

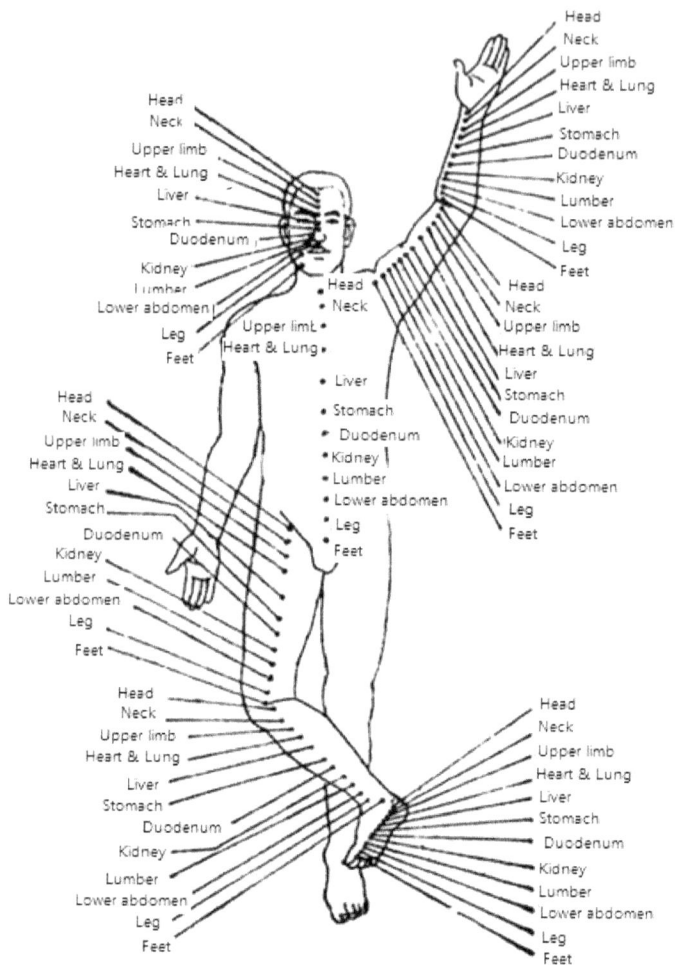

Head
Neck
Upper limb
Heart & Lung
Liver
Stomach
Duodenum
Kidney
Lumber
Lower abdomen
Leg
Feet

Head
Neck
Upper limb
Heart & Lung
Liver
Stomach
Duodenum
Kidney
Lumber
Lower abdomen
Leg
Feet

Head
Neck
Upper limb
Heart & Lung
Liver
Stomach
Duodenum
Kidney
Lumber
Lower abdomen
Leg
Feet

Head
Neck
Upper limb
Heart & Lung
Liver
Stomach
Duodenum
Kidney
Lumber
Lower abdomen
Leg
Feet

Head
Neck
Upper limb
Heart & Lung
Liver
Stomach
Duodenum
Kidney
Lumber
Lower abdomen
Leg
Feet

Head
Neck
Upper limb
Heart & Lung
Liver
Stomach
Duodenum
Kidney
Lumber
Lower abdomen
Leg
Feet

Head
Neck
Upper limb
Heart & Lung
Liver
Stomach
Duodenum
Kidney
Lumber
Lower abdomen
Leg
Feet

Holographic chart of acupuncture points

Figure 48. Holographic chart of acupuncture points.[157]

Another example is the second and the fifth Metacarpal bone holographic acupuncture.

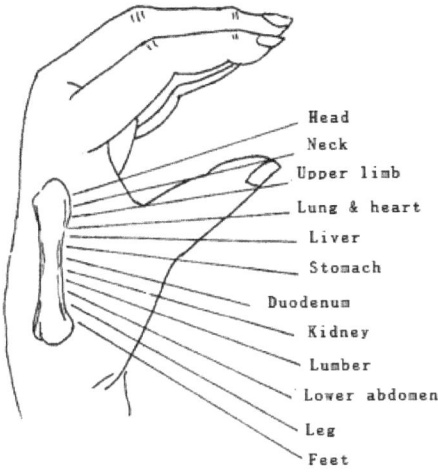

Figure 49. Holographic chart for second metacarpal bone.[158]

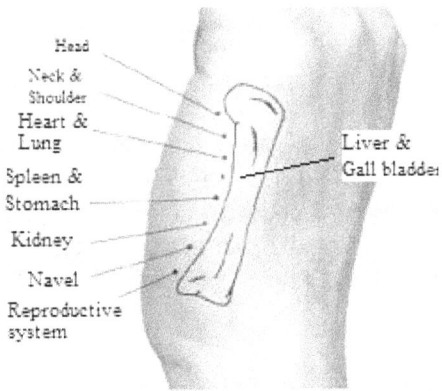

Figure 50. Holographic chart for the fifty metacarpal bone.[159]

(20)   Feng Ning-Han Nine-place Acupuncture style (冯宁汉九宫针法)

This acupuncture style was developed by Professor Feng Ning-Han. The idea came from the book "*Zhen Jiu Da Cheng*". In treatment, choose and find the sick point on the body first. This point will be the middle point (Middle Palace). Then select eight other points around the middle point (so called nine palaces), about 2-5 cm from the middle point. Insert the first needle on the middle point. For the remaining needles, insert them in the sequence of upper palace first, then lower palace, left, then right, upper-left, upper-right, lower-left, and finally lower-right (Figure 51). The sequence can be understand as a clock: middle needle first, then insert the needle at 0 am (12 pm), then 6 am, then 3 am, then 9 pm, then 1.5 am, then 10.5 pm, then 4.5 am, and finally 7.5 am.

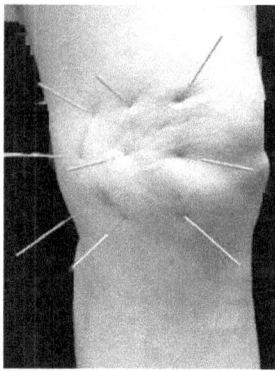

Figure 51. Acupuncture illustration of Nine-palace acupuncture style.[160]

There is no need to manipulate the needle to induce Deqi sensation. We do acupuncture on the lower limb (to nourish or balance the Jing, e.g. micro essence material), the middle body (to nourish the Qi) and the head (to nourish the Spirit), no matter if the disease is mild or severe, and no matter if the diseases are caused by inner or outer reasons.[161]

Zhao Mei (赵梅) (2012) [162] treated 100 cases of prolapse of lumbar intervertebral disc by using the Nine-palace acupuncture (Deqi session was induced), plus traditional acupuncture points, herbal paste, TDP lamp, middle-frequency treatment machine, and an ion-inducing machine. After the treatment, 57 cases were cured, 35 cases were much improved, and only 8 cases had no improvement. To cure, as little as 10 days and as many as 20 sessions were needed.

(21)   Guan Zhen-Zai Nine-Palace Acupuncture style (管正斋九宫针法)

This style of acupuncture was developed by Dr. Guan Zhen-Zai.[163] This way of acupuncture is similar to the above style, but is mostly used on the spine. It requires the retention of needles for 30 min and the manipulation of needles three times during the session. It is said that this technique of acupuncture works mostly for diseases that are related to disorders of the spine: various spondylarthritis, spinal trauma, injury of supraspinal ligament, cervical spondylopathy, lumbar hyperosteogeny, thoracic vertebrae hyperosteogeny, prolapse of lumbar intervertebral disc, lumbar sprain, lumbar degeneration.

Cheng GL (2008) [164] treated 526 cases of prolapse of lumbar intervertebral disc with the Nine-palace acupuncture (Deqi session was induced), plus traditional acupuncture points and cupping. After treatment, 35 cases were cured, 251 cases were much improved, and 240 cases were improved. The authors did not report how many sessions were needed.

There is another acupuncture style called Nine palace-twelve way style, which was developed and used by Dr. Yin Xue-Chen.[165, 166] It uses nine special needles for the treatment.[33]

(22)   Along-spine acupuncture style (脊针针法)

There are acupuncture points along the spine, independent of the traditional Jia Ji point. The style used here is called Ji needle acupuncture (Along spine acupuncture). The acupuncture points are on 0.5 body cun on the both side of the spinal spinous process, from cervical spine (7 pairs), thoracic (12 pairs), and lumber (5 pairs), to the sacral spine (4 pairs).
The points in the cervical pairs work for the diseases in the head, face, neck and upper limbs, such as nerve pain, spondylosis, tonsillitis or stiff shoulder.

The points in the thoracic pairs work for diseases in the upper limb (thoracic pair 1 to 3), such as shoulder pain, cough, asthma, chest pain; in the chest (thoracic pair 4 -9), such as palpitation, angina pectoris, stomach pain; and in the stomach (thoracic pair 10 – 12), such as pain in liver region, biliary colic, biliary ascariasis.

The points in the lumber pairs work for diseases in the stomach, lower lumber and lower limb, such as stomach pain, abdomen bloating, ap-

---

[33] Detailed data is not available.

pendicitis, enteritis, pain in the leg, paralysis, and pain in the lumber-sacral region.

The points in the sacral pairs work for diseases in the urinary and reproductive systems, such as impotency, spermatorrhea, enuresis, prolapse of the anus, uterine prolapse, dysmenorrhea, amenorrhea, paralysis in leg, pain in leg, or lumbosacral strain.

The acupuncture points are chosen based on where pain is felt by pressing, or on the known connection of the anatomic relationship between the level of spine and the organs connected via nerves.

Acupuncture on spine pairs requires Deqi sensation and is usually combined with body acupuncture treatment.

3. Local acupuncture styles for local diseases

(1) A Shi point acupuncture (阿是穴疗法)

A Shi point acupuncture belongs to traditional Chinese acupuncture. It is one of the ways to select acupuncture points for treatment. We press the body surface to find the painful spot, then to stimulate the painful spot for treatment. It is called the A Shi point because the patient would yell out "A" when pressing this point.

The A Shi point can be stimulated by acupuncture needle, by fingers (called finger press acupressure), or with electric machines, such as TENS, Hans machine, etc. For diseases in the muscle (soft tissue), such treatments apparently work pretty well.

If the local disease is on the skin, the acupuncturist can just insert the needles on and around the skin lesion. The number of the needles can be as little as four needles (Yang ci acupuncture), or as many as more than ten needles. The needles can evenly distributed on and around the skin lesion (branch needles), or can be one circle or even two circles around the skin lesion.

For severe muscle diseases, the acupuncturist may also use a small tool, called Needle-knife, which is inserted into the skin to losen the stiff tissue under the skin (the Small Needle-knife technique).

Sometimes, the acupuncturist may also pouch the painful spot to release some drops of blood, and then cover the spot with a cupping cup (called Bleeding Cupping technique).

All of these therapies indicate that a local disease can also be treated with local stimulation, without consideration of traditional meridian diagnosis or TCM organ diagnosis.

(2) Release point acupuncture (反阿是穴疗法)

Release point acupuncture (反阿是穴) is the opposite style to A Shi point style. It was developed by Dr. Zhang Wen-Bing and Dr. Huo Ze-Jun.[167]

This style of acupuncture is also mostly used for the treatment of soft tissue damage. The release point means that, upon pressing some point on the muscle, the original pain in the affected muscle becomes released or disappears, although under the Release point, there is somehow pain or discomfort upon being pressed.

The location of the Release point is opposite to the A Shi point but they are basically on the same group of muscles. If the A Shi point is located on the starting point of the muscle, the Release point is on the middle or the end of the muscle. If the A Shi point is located on the middle of the muscle, the Release point is on the starting or end part of the muscle group. If the A Shi point is on the end point of the muscle, the Release point is on the starting part of the muscle.

There is usually tightness under the Release point. Upon pressing the Release point and letting the patient move the affected limb or joint, the patient would feel much release of the pain on the original pain spot. This is a very important way to find the Release point.

Similar to the treatment of the A Shi point, the Release point can also be stimulated with acupuncture needle, finger press, point injection, or fire needle, and so on.

Some acupuncturists[168] believe that the use of this method works better for acute soft tissue damage. For chronic and repeated soft tissue damage, it can be used as an alternative choice.

(3) Trigger point (扳机点疗法)

The concept of the Trigger point was firstly described comprehensively by Dr. Janet G. Travell. A Trigger point is a spot on the surface of the body.[169] Touching it could cause pain, cause a local muscle twitch, or cause pain in another place (referred pain). A patient may have more than 2 Trigger points and the Trigger points can be located on the primary pain spot, near it, or far away from it.

On the Trigger point, the acupuncturist can usually find a painful knob or tight muscle mass. Once the Trigger point is identified, then the acupuncturist can use acupuncture needles, point injection, or electric stimulation (such as TENS) for the treatment.

It should be pointed out that the Trigger point is not at all the acupuncture point, the A Shi point or the Release point noted above.[170]

(4) Liu Nong-Yu Sinew acupuncture (刘农虞筋针疗法)

Tendon acupuncture was developed by Dr. Liu Nong-Yu.[171] It is mostly used for the treatment of soft tissue diseases. We select places about 2 to 3 cun from a painful spot or knob along the affected tendon as acupuncture points, e.g. along-tendon diagnosis. There is no need to have any TCM or meridian diagnosis. The needle is inserted shallowly (penetrating subcutaneously under the skin, not in the muscle layer). The technique only stimulates the membrane of the tendon. There should be no apparent pain or strong discomfort during acupuncture. It is reported that at the first treatment, the pain level can be reduced by more than 50%. Generally only one to three needles are needed for each session.

Tendon acupuncture is used for treatment of the following diseases: acute neck spasm, cervical spondylosis, intercostal neuralgia, acute lumbar sprain, lumbar muscle degeneration, periarthritis of shoulder, post-stroke shoulder pain, tennis elbow, carpal tunnel syndrome, loose tendon in the finger, trigger finger, soft tissue damage, heel pain, gout, and so on. For these diseases, the more pain there is, the better the healing effect is.

II. Characteristics of current acupuncture styles

1. Acupuncture points to be stimulated

In current acupuncture practice, not all the acupuncture points belong to the traditional meridian system. Points could also be chosen according to Holographic theory, the Eight Diagram theory, the Mirror theory, the Extra Point system, the nerve distribution zones and the positive point on the body (Table 1).

Table 1. The ways of choosing acupuncture points

Meridian-based acupuncture style	Traditional acupuncture style (Textbook acupuncture)
	Time-circle acupuncture
	Tan Wu-Bian Balancing acupuncture
	Liu Ji-Ling new one-needle acupuncture
	Zhang Xian-Chen Hand-Foot Three-needle acupuncture
	Flying acupuncture
	Zhao Wu-Rong Flying acupuncture
	Li Jin-Niu Five-element acupuncture
	Ma Xiao-Ping Five-element acupuncture
	Yangming Five-element acupuncture
	Mang acupuncture style
	Guo Zhi-Chen Eight-point acupuncture
	Pan Xiao-Chuan Classical acupuncture
	Korea Sha-Am Five-element acupuncture
	Korea Li Ji-Ma Four-diagram acupuncture
	Nora Five-element acupuncture
	Some Japanese acupuncture
	Bo Zhi-Yun abdominal acupuncture style

Holographic theory-based acupuncture style	Most kinds of scalp acupuncture styles
	Facial acupuncture style
	Eye acupuncture style
	Nose acupuncture style
	Mouth acupuncture style
	Tongue acupuncture style
	Ren-zhong acupuncture style
	Some Palm acupuncture styles
	Foot acupuncture style
Mirror theory-based acupuncture style	Wang Wen-Yuan Balancing acupuncture
	Tan Wu-Bian Balancing acupuncture
	Li Bai-Song Eight-words acupuncture
	Chen Zhao Crane-Pine Yi Xue acupuncture
	Ke Shang-Zhi Distance-meridian acupressure therapy
Eight Diagram or Nine palace theory-based acupuncture style	Navel Eight-diagram style
	Abdominal Eight-diagram style
	Liu Bing-Quan Eight-diagram scalp style
	Chen Zhao Crane-Pine Yi Xue acupuncture
	Peng Jing-Shan eye Eight-diagram acupuncture
	Feng Ning-Han Nine-Palace acupuncture style
	Guan Zhen-Zai Nine-Palace acupuncture
	Yin Xue-Chen Nine-Palace acupuncture
Extra point-based acupuncture style	Dong Jing-Chang Extra point acupuncture style

	Han Wen-Zhi One-needle acupuncture style
	Zhang Xin-Shu Wrist-ankle acupuncture
Nerve distribution zones	Along-spine acupuncture style
Pain spot-based acupuncture style	A Shi acupuncture
	Release point acupuncture
	Trigger point acupuncture
	Liu Nong-Yu Tendon acupuncture
	Western Medical acupuncture

2. Diagnosis directing the selection of the acupuncture point

Acupuncture points can be selected according to meridian diagnosis, traditional TCM organ, Qi-Blood diagnosis, Four-Jiao space diagnosis (the Upper Jiao, Middle Jiao, Lower Jiao and Outer Jiao,四焦辩证), the Four-region diagnosis (四象辩证, e.g. the corresponding location of the diseases), the Four Diagram diagnosis (四局辩证) and the location diagnosis (such as for the treatment of headache, choosing the corresponding "head" point in various Holographic acupuncture systems), or by just touching the local tissue for positive points.

3. Steady point versus dynamic points

Acupuncture points can be steady, such as in the traditional acupuncture systems. The points can also be dynamic. This means that the points show up only during disease conditions, such as the positive reactive point in Tan Wu Bian Balancing acupuncture, Li Bai-Song Eight-words acupuncture, A Shi acupuncture, Release acupuncture style, Trigger point acupuncture, and Liu's Sinew acupuncture. They target the positive reactive points requiring stimulation. The points do not exist in normal and healthy body condition.

4. Accuracy of acupuncture points

Some acupuncture styles require very accurate locations of the acupuncture spots, such as the Bo Zhi-Yun acupuncture style. Some do not require so much accuracy, such as various Eight-Diagram and Nine-Palace acupuncture styles, in which the acupuncture works under the condition that the needles are inserted in the correct diagram (or in a zone). Some acupuncture styles do not need precise acupuncture points, but need the precise positive points (Tan Wu-Bian Balancing acupuncture, Li Bai-Song Eight-words acupuncture, the A Shi points, the Release point, the Trigger points and the Liu Nong-Yu Sinew acupuncture).

5. Depth of needle insertion

The needle used in treatment can be very deep in the body, such as the Mang acupuncture style, in which the needle can be inserted into the body (horizontally) for more than 30 cm; or the Han Wen-Zhi One-needle acupuncture style, in which most of the needles are inserted for 2 to 3 body cun. The needle can also be very shallow, such as in some Japanese acupuncture styles, in which the needles are inserted into the skin for only 1-2 mm. Some Chinese shallow acupuncture styles insert needle at least to the hypodermis layer and aim to induce the Deqi sensation too.[86] Some acupuncture styles insert the needle only in the subcutaneous layer, not into the muscle, such as Liu Ji-Ling new one-needle acupuncture, Fu Zhong-Hua subcutaneous acupuncture, Bo Zhi-Yun abdominal acupuncture, Wrist-ankle acupuncture, and Liu Nong-Yu Sinew acupuncture.

6. Intensity of treatment stimulation

The intensity of the acupuncture stimulation can be very strong, such as in the Dr. Shi Xue-Ming style of acupuncture, in which the needle needs to touch the nerve, in Ke Shang-Zhi Distance-meridian acupressure therapy, in which skin might be pressed hard to blue-purple color (bruise), in the Li Bai-Song Eight-words acupuncture and in the Zhang Xian-Chen Hand-Foot Three-needle acupuncture style. The needle feeling can also be very mild or almost nothing, such as in the Liu Ji-Ling new one-needle acupuncture, Bo Zhi-Yun Abdominal acupuncture, Eight-Diagram abdominal acupuncture, Wrist-ankle acupuncture,

Liu Nong-Yu Sinew acupuncture, or in some Japanese acupuncture styles.

7. Healing efficiency of acupuncture styles

This is a very sensitive question in discussion. The answer might not be proper if there is no direct comparative study with the experts in each acupuncture style in the study. But each acupuncture style could have its own favorite and relatively not-so-favorite disease spectrum. For example, the various scalp acupuncture styles are commonly used for the treatment of nerve-affected disease, or brain-originated diseases, such as stroke, chorea festinans, paralysis, Bell's palsy, migraine, child cerebral palsy, supranuclear paralysis, epilepsy, dystaxia, epileptiform neuralgia, and sciatic pain, though it is also used for the treatment of other kinds of diseases.

Bo Zhi-Yun Abdominal acupuncture works relatively better for inside organ-related diseases, whereas various Positive point-related local acupuncture styles (such as A Shi point acupuncture, Release point acupuncture, Trigger point acupuncture, Tendon acupuncture, Fu Zhong-Hua subcutaneous acupuncture, etc.) work relatively better for local muscle-tendon originating diseases, such as shoulder pain, tennis elbow, carpal tunnel syndrome, lower back pain, and various muscle spasm (including sciatic pain).

Some acupuncture styles work better for acute pain than for chronic pain, such as the Wang Wen-Yuan Balancing acupuncture style. Some other acupuncture styles can work for even severe conditions (such as stroke), such as the Shi Xue-Ming Enhancing acupuncture style. Some acupuncture styles even work better for time-related disease (e.g. the onset of the disease is with fixed time of the day, the month, or the season), such as various Time-circle acupuncture styles.

For us as acupuncturists, we need to know the advantages and disadvantages of the various acupuncture styles. The acupuncture style to be applied is not only based on the nature of the diseases, but also on the patient. If the patient cannot tolerate much pain, we may consider the Zhang Xin-Shu Wrist-ankle acupuncture, the Liu Nong-Yu Sinew acupuncture, the Bo Zhi-Yun Abdominal acupuncture style, the Eight-diagram abdominal acupuncture, or the Qi Yong Navel acupuncture.

8. Whole body acupuncture versus local acupuncture

One of the characteristics of Chinese medicine is that it emphasizes viewing disease from a whole body perspective. For this, acupuncturists believe that a local disease could influence the whole body, and that the treatment from the whole body aspect could also help to solve the local disease (such as carpal tunnel syndrome or ankle strain) and the whole body acupuncture would work much better than a local acupuncture.

This view may not always be true.

That a local can influence the whole and the whole can also influence the local is a philosophic idea. In practice, we need to know how much influence there might be. The local disease may or may not clearly influence the whole body and cause detectable structural and functional change. A structural and functional change in the whole body may or may not influence a local part of the body very much either. For example, a traffic accident on one street in the city of Edmonton may not dramatically influence the traffic of the whole city. A sick person with a whole body disease, such as hypertension, coronary heart disease, still has functional normal movement of their arms and legs.

In acupuncture practice, this means that some local diseases can be cured with a local treatment, such as A Shi point acupuncture, Release point acupuncture, Liu Nong-Yu Sinew acupuncture, and Wrist-ankle acupuncture. The acupuncturist does not really need to test the Five-element nature of the patients, or to solve the local pain or swelling by adjusting the pulse. Under such local pain, especially for a chronic pain, the pulse may not be clearly abnormal. Also, if the patient also has other chronic diseases, the pulse would be too variable to allow clear diagnosis. If so, the adjustment of the pulse would be difficult and it tends to fail in the treatment. In such instances, we have tried traditional acupuncture but the patient still felt a high level of pain. After, we used the TENS (or fire needle technique, or bleeding-cupping) locally, and the pain subsided much more.

III. Acupuncture research

There are many ways to practice acupuncture. The acupuncture point can be chosen in different places; the points may be chosen from meridians, or not; the number of needles used can be only one or more than 10, 20 or even 30; the depth of the needle can be as shallow as just into the epidermis, or it can go into the hypodermis, deep into muscle or even touch the bone membrane; the Deqi sensation is required in some acupuncture styles, while it is prevented in some other styles.

There are still questions that the acupuncture researchers must answer:

First, are all or some of the acupuncture styles actually a placebo effect? Given the large variation in acupuncture methodology, it is very easy to suspect that acupuncture might be just a placebo effect.

The most questionable acupuncture style is the Nora Five-element acupuncture style, in which it is said that the most important part of the treatment is the good relationship between the acupuncturist and their patients, and that the influence of the acupuncture technique is less important. Such characteristics are very rare in Chinese styles of acupuncture.

Another questionable style is Japanese acupuncture in which the needles are inserted very shallowly into the skin (1 mm).[62] The healing effect of very shallow acupuncture, such as some Japanese acupuncture styles, has been questioned long time ago by some Chinese acupuncture masters.[172] Not many acupuncture studies have been done in Japan. In one review (1978-2006),[173] the reviewers could find only 57 papers on the subject, among which only 20 are full papers and the remaining 37 are case reports. Conditions examined were headache (12 trials), chronic lower back pain (9 trials), rheumatoid arthritis (8 trials), temporomandibular dysfunction (8 trials), katakori (8 trials) and others (12 trials). Applying the 5-point Jadad quality assessment scoring style, the mean score was 1.5 ± 1.3 (SD). The reviewers concluded that "there is limited evidence that acupuncture is more effective than no treatment."

This is very strange. In fact, even if we questioned whether the Chinese style of acupuncture is just a placebo effect, the researchers have to admit that the healing effect of acupuncture done in the hands is almost always significantly higher than no treatment (though it may not be higher than in placebo groups). We are therefore strongly interested in knowing whether the shallow-inserted needle acupuncture of the Japanese style is mostly a placebo effect.

The second big question for acupuncture researchers is that it seems that anywhere on the body can be stimulated as an acupuncture point for the treatment of disease. Although, for a given disease, we still needs to stimulate specific points, or regions, or zones of the body for the treatment. For example, for the treatment of headache, we can stimulate some spots on the head, the face, the eye, the nose, the feet, the hands, the arm, the stomach, or the navel, but in each region, we still needs to follow some rule to find the proper spots to stimulate. The function of some points can be explained by meridian theory, but some cannot.

The third question regards the relative advantages and disadvantages of each style of acupuncture. Each of acupuncture style should be compared with textbook acupuncture. The recommended diseases that should be compared are the following:

(1) nonspecific lower back pain;
(2) migraine;
(3) IBS;
(4) facial paralysis;
(5) post-operative nausea/vomit (acupuncture starts 30 min before operation and lasts to the end of the surgery);
(6) post-stroke paralysis or post-stroke depression;

All of these disease conditions are within the dominant advantage pattern of Chinese acupuncture.

In the study of acupuncture, it is better to separate Western medical acupuncture from the Chinese style of acupuncture. It has been recognized that there exists such Western styles of acupuncture that use needle for treatment but do not follow the traditional meridian diagnosis or TCM organ diagnosis to guide the choice of acupuncture points. Any reviewers should be aware of this fact and indicate which acupuncture style is reviewed in their review articles.

In the acupuncture comparison study, the exact practical procedures for the given style of acupuncture should be followed and are best performed by the expert in that style. For example, in the study of Nora Five-element acupuncture, the acupuncture should be performed as once a week for 6-8 sessions. However, if we are comparing that style to the Chinese style of acupuncture, then the acupuncture should still be performed once a week for 6 or 8 sessions, with 2 days break before each course for a total of 6 to 8 weeks. In this way, we can compare the healing effect within the same treatment period (6 or 8 weeks), and also the same sessions (6 to 8 sessions).

The most difficult question is the mechanism of the acupuncture. Any theory needs not only to explain one style of acupuncture, but, at best, be able to explain all of the acupuncture styles.

There are several hypotheses regarding the mechanism of acupuncture. With a big picture of current acupuncture styles in mind, it is easy to find that Blood vessel theory, the Nerve reflection theory and the Fibro-membrane theory might work for the local acupuncture styles (A Shi point acupuncture, Release point acupuncture, Trigger point acupuncture, Liu Nong-Yu Sinew acupuncture), the Fu Zhong-Hua subcutaneous acupuncture and the Wrist-ankle acupuncture, but it is difficult to explain all the Holographic theory-based and the Eight-diagram theory-based acupuncture styles.

Currently, it seems very difficult to find a single theory to explain the mechanism of all styles of acupuncture.[174, 175, 176]

It has been pointed[175] out that the meridian is a complex network structure in the body. It consists of at least seven kinds of bio-network structures, such as the collagenous fiber network, the polysaccharide/ aquagel fibre net, and the tissue fluid transportation network, etc. The acupuncture point is imbedded in the soft connective tissue. Meridian phenomenon is the holistic biological phenomenon of these net structures. It might be that studying acupuncture mechanisms is as difficult as the study of telepathy. The mechanism of acupuncture might involve the transfer of information, which is another parameter of the concrete physical material world, besides the material, space location, time, and so on.

Conclusion

The aim of this paper is to supply basic information about various acupuncture techniques currently in practice, not only in Western countries, but also in China. We need to know that the textbook acupuncture style is only one style in use, and that it is used mostly in Western countries or in China. This is simply because this style was introduced in textbook form to many people. It does not mean that it is the best style of acupuncture, though the textbook has also introduced some other way of acupuncture, such as Time-circle acupuncture and Eight-diagram acupuncture, etc.

Currently in the US, for example, the most used acupuncture styles are textbook acupuncture, Dong's extraordinary point acupuncture, Five-element acupuncture, Tang's Balancing acupuncture, some Japanese acupuncture, Korea acupuncture, and Western medical acupuncture.[177] Acupuncturists must know the realities of the acupuncture profession and know different ways of acupuncture, so as to apply the proper style of acupuncture to each patient.

For acupuncture research, we may still have a long way to go to under-stand the precise mechanism of acupuncture, but this should not pre-vent researchers from finding out if acupuncture really has its own unique healing effect, beyond the placebo effect.

Our Publications

- More Than Acupuncture (book)
- Acupuncture for Emergencies (book)
- Acupuncture Styles in Current Practice (book)
- What We Can Learn from Acupuncture Research in Western Countries (book)
- Does Nora Five-element Acupuncture Depend mostly on Psychological Effect? (book)
- Current Opinions on Shanghan Lun
- Current opinions on Classical Formulas

Books are available in amazon.com

References

[1] Liang FR. Acupuncture- Textbook for New century National Chinese Medicine University. China Traditional Chinese Medicine Press, Beijing, China. 2005.

[2] Sun GJ. Acupuncture- Textbook for Chinese Medicine University. Shanghai science and Technology Press, Shanghai, China.1997.

[3] Qiu ML, Zhang SC. Acupuncture- Textbook for Chinese Medicine University. Shanghai science and Technology Press, Shanghai, China. 1985.

[4] Deng LY, Gan YJ, He Shuhui, Ji XP, Li Yang, Wang RF, Wang WJ, Wang XT, Xu HZ, Xue XL and Yuan JL. Chinese Acupuncture and Moxibustion. Foreign Languages Press. Beijing, China. 2012

[5] Steve C. Giovanni M. The Practice of Chinese Medicine. Second edition. Churchill Livingstone, Elsevier. 2008

[6] Chen Su, Huang FX, Ke ZL, Yang ZG. Treatment various diseases with unique and special acupuncture points. Fujiang science and Technology Press, China. 1985.

[7] He GX. Precise importance and usefulness of special and unique acupuncture points founded in and out of China. Beijing science and Technology Press, Beijing, China.

[8] Li QZ. Zi Wu Circulation – Alive Fossil in Traditional Chinese Medicine. www.epochtimes.com/b5/16/2/9/n4636499.htm

[9] Qigong Practitioner Network. Zi Yu Circulation Chart. www.qgren.com/qigong/lilun/384.shtml

[10] Amy K. Five element chart. https://www.amykuretsky.com/blog/the-five-elements

[11] Kang CQ. Clinic Application of Zi Wu Time Circulation in Acupuncture. www.wfas.org.cn/lunwen/wfas10/201109/3346.html

[12] Guan ZH, Ding LL, Guo CP, Ye J, Yi R. Clinical application of Zi Wu Time Circulation Chart. J Chin Integr Med. 2003; 1(4):314-316

[13] Zhou GT. Discussion about the Zi Wu Time Circulation with Professor Cao Yi Ming. Tianjin J Traditional Chinese Med. 2004; 21(1):4-6

[14] Li ZQ. Talk about Ling Gui Eight methods by Master Ni Hai Xia. http://blog.sina.com.cn/s/blog_ead9736c0102wix1.html

[15] Peng ZF. Re-question about the Earth branch of Zi Wu Circulation. www.tcmforum.com/forum2.php?forumID=522

[16] Li L. Dialectically Thinking about Acupuncture with Zi Wu Circulation Theory. http://cntcm.39kf.com/shtml/2317-b-8.shtml

[17] Health DIY website. Argument about Zi Wu Circulation: A phenomenon that was not Mentioned in either book Nei Jing or book Shang Han Lun. http://yannan.byethost5.com/health/health04.htm

[18] Yuan J, Li M, Zhang SZ, Wang YM, Ning P, Sun X, Kang GH. Clinic study of ischemic cerebrovascular disease with acupuncture using Zi Wu circulation and TCM diagnosis. Hebei J Traditional Chinese Med. 2014;11:1669-1671

[19] Liu DR, Hao SF, Liu ZY. Clinic observation of acupuncture treatment of cerebral infarction with "Na Jia method of Zi Wu circulation" . Chinese Acup & Moxi. 2009; 29(5): 353-356

[20] Han ZX, Liu YG, Wei JL. Influence of "Na Jia method of Zi Wu circulation" on the treatment of cerebral infarction. Chinese Acup & Moxi. 2008; 28(12): 865-868

[21] Zhang ZX. Clinic observation on 30 cases of insomnia treated with the acupuncture and with Na Jia method and Fei Teng Eight methods of Zi Wu Time circulation. Clinical J Chinese Med. 2013;(6): 47-48

[22] Guan ZH, Yi R, Ye J, Ding LL, Zhu XY, Guo CP. Study of influence of initiation of acupuncture points with Zi Wu circulation on myocardial ischemia level in stroke patients. Chinese Acup & Moxi. 2005; 25(11): 823-824

[23] Zhang JH, Shao ZL, Fei XY, Jiang Y, Yang SL. Influence of Zi Wu time circulation acupuncture on immune function of chronic hepatitis C patients. Chinese Acup & Moxi. 2004; 24(10): 693-694

[24] Wang Wen Yuan Balancing Acupuncture Technique. http://www.100md.com/index/0h/d1/0a/16/index.htm

[25] Strinkers. Characteristics of Tang's Balancing Acupuncture system. http://bbs.iiyi.com/thread-2548630-1.html

[26] Si Yuan Balance Method Acupuncture. www.siyuanbalance.com/

[27] Eight-word Acupuncture Therapy. www.360doc.com/content/10/0818/09/840524_47041342.shtml

[28] Xian Zai lay Buddhist. Eight-word Acupuncture Chart. http://blog.sina.com.cn/s/blog_6383a68a0102e3sg.html

[29] Yang's style of acupuncture: Dr. Chen Zhao: The first ancestor of Yi Acupuncture. http://sjzlu.blog.sohu.com/130194866.html

[30] Ikegadad. How many methods in the Crane-pine Yi Xue Acupuncture of Dr. Chen Zhao?. http://www.sanwen8.com/p/u4fectdo.html

[31] Jiu Ji-ling. Liu Ji Ling New One-needle Acupuncture. https://v.qq.com/x/page/v0191de3sdh.html

[32] Acupuncture-Tuina massage website. Learn New One-needle Acupuncture from Zero Knowledge of Acupuncture. http://wtoutiao.com/p/6e5eHWU.html

[33] Website of Five-element Blooming. New explanation about Dr. Zhang's Hand-Feet Three-needle Acupuncture. http://www.360doc.com/content/13/0526/09/11980212_288236524.shtml

[34] Website of Colorful Cloud Racing behind Bamboo. Treatment of pain on neck, shoulder, lumber and leg, with Hand-feet Three-needle Acupuncture. http://www.360doc.com/content/11/0606/21/533142_122106761.shtml

[35] Blog of One-needle-one-world-599. Jin Three-needle Acupuncture Therapy. http://baike.baidu.com/view/640926.htm

[36] FSN World. Floating Acupuncture Outline: Medicine needs new battle field. http://www.fuzhen.com.cn/xnew.asp?nid=868

[37] Tao JL, Fu ZH, Zhang HR. The Analysis with Mechanism of Fu's Subcutaneous Needling. Lishizhen Med Materia Medica Res. 2014;25(12): 3006-3008

[38] He QT. Cited. Misunderstanding on FNS Acupuncture (2nd part). http://www.haodf.com/zhuanjiaguandian/drheqingtao_1458384285.htm

[39] Zhao WR. Treatment of multiple diseases with Flying Acupuncture therapy. People's Health Press. 2011.

[40] Li XL: Inheritor of the Fold Unique Acupuncture "Flying Acupuncture". zy.china.com.cn

[41] China newspaper of traditional Chinese Medicine: South Ling Chen's Flying Acupuncture. http://www.wujue.com/zljs/zljs/zhenci/201104/42664.html

[42] Li JN, Huo SK, Qiao JL. Five Element Nourishing-Counteracting Acupuncture Technique. J Sichuan of TCM. 2009;27(2):120-121

[43] Ma XP. Clinic Application of Depleting-South and Nourishing-North Acupuncture. Jiangsu J TCM. 1990, 8:25-26

[44] Ding ZX, Jin HY, Zhang YZ. Application of Five-element theory in Acupuncture practice. 8th Conference on Neijing studies. China Association of TCM. 2006. 252-255

[45] Ding LL, Ma QJ, Ma JH. Clinical observation on the treatment of 60 cases of simple obesity with Yangming Five-element style of acupuncture. Clinical J Chinese Med. 2016;8(23):123-125

[46] Mang style of acupuncture. http://baike.baidu.com/view/5335366.htm

[47] Beijing Yao Medicine Hospital. Demonstration the needles used in the Mang style of acupuncture. http://bj.dekunyy.com/html/yaoyi_488_1.html

[48] Zhou Xin. Experience after using Mang acupuncture for the treatment of post-stroke syndrome. http://blog.39.net/zhouxin54/a_16530628.html

[49] Gate website for Dong's extraordinary acupuncture system. Demonstration of Mang acupuncture by Prof. Li Guo Zheng. https://www.youtube.com/watch?v=XXUGN31CBIw

[50] Demonstration of Mang Acupuncture. https://www.youtube.com/watch?v=-ASKxsCJCGo

[51] New Yuan Qi College. Online Class for Guo's Eight -Points Style of Acupuncture. http://hopeyoubetter.blogspot.ca/2014/11/blog-post_41.html

[52] H Zhu Q. Pan Xiao Chuan theory of medicine: Self-harmonization system. http://www.360doc.com/content/16/0808/11/11285146_581635215.shtml

[53] Classic Chinese Medicine Website: Pan Xiao Chuan theory of Chinese Medicine: Topic on Chinese medicine technique. http://clasictcm.com/archives/257

[54] Pan Shi-Nan: Sharing the learning of the Acupuncture Zhen-Ling of the Classical TCM by Teacher Pan Xiao Chuan. https://www.youtube.com/watch?v=e8ALXACZsfA

[55] Youn YS. Korean SHA-AM acupuncture introduction. Tianjin J TCM. 2010; 27(3):259-260

[56] Jin CY. Consideration of Taiji acupuncture of Korea Medicine. J Med and Pharmacy of Chinese Minorities. 2009;9:9-40

[57] Old Generation Medicine Collection: Five Element Acupuncture: A very old and mysterious style of acupuncture. http://www.laozongyi.com/zhongyi/284197.html

[58] Yin Shui Zai. First review of lecture for Five Element acupuncture. http://www.360doc.com/content/16/0614/13/20849286_567684411.shtml

[59] Zi Sou. Notebook for 《Guidance for Five Element Acupuncture》. http://blog.sina.com.cn/s/blog_7da0ca120102vwto.html

[60] Notebook for Study of TCM. The five personal characters in the Five Element acupuncture. http://zhong1.org/2228.html

[61] Liang Ni. Theoretical discussion of the treatment of post-stroke depression with Five-element acupuncture. Chinese J Integrative Med Cardio/Cerebrovas Dis. 2015;13(17):1958-1960

[62] Xiao YZ, Zhang LJ, Huang QX. Overall introduction of famous acupuncture styles in Japan. International J TCM. 2011;33(5):461-464

[63] Zhi Fa Medical Thesis Website. Overview of contribution to acupuncture by Japanese. http://www.zhifayixue.com/zhongyaolunwen/425.html

[64] Chinese Traditional Culture Website. Brief Introduction of Japanese Acupuncture. http://www.100md.com/Html/Dir0/15/16/23.htm

[65] Kiiko Matsumoto. Diagnosis in Kiiko Matsumoto Style (KMS) Acupuncture. http://www.pacificcollege.edu/sites/default/files/PS2016Notes/3/KobyleckaM_PS2016_SaturdayAM_Handout.pdf

[66] Kiiko Matsumoto. Fertility Support. https://bconroytc.wikispaces.com/Fertility+Support+-+Kiiko+Matsumoto+Japanese+Style

[67] He XG, Li X. Clinical observation on the effect of Waking-up-clear-mind acupuncture therapy in the treatment of coma patients due to brain trauma. World Health Digest. 2012; 47: 71-72

[68] Shen PF, Shi XM. Evaluation of antihypertensive effect of acupuncture essential hypertension by ambulatory blood pressure monitorin. Liaoning J TCM. 2010;37(9):1802-1803

[69] Yu NN, Chen ZL, Huo Y. The inner meaning and key points in application of "Fei Jing Zou Qi" acupuncture technique. J Shanghai Acupuncture and Moxibution. 2014, 33(4):

[70] Lou SK. *Ci Fa Jiu Fa Xue*. China Traditional Chinese Medicine Publishing House. Beijing. 2003: 81-83

[71] Wang FC. *Ci Fa Jiu Fa Xue*. China Traditional Chinese Medicine Publishing House. Beijing. 2009:55

[72] Chen YL, Zheng KS. Zhang TH, *et al.* "Jie Qi Tong Jing" acupuncture technique. Shanghai J TCM. 2001; 35(6):24-25

[73] Yang ZY. Introduction of "Xing Qi" acupuncture technique by Dr. Li Yu-Lin. J Tianjin University of TCM. 1982; 1(00): 41-43

[74] Xu JM. Wang CH. Discussion of the four ways of "Fei Jing Zou Qi". J Shanghai Acupuncture and Moxibustion. 2008;27(7): 46-47

[75] Wu XF. Report of the treatment of 2 cases of Guillain-Barre Syndrome with big continuous meridian acupuncture technique. J Zhejiang University of TCM. 2016; 40(6):288-490

[76] Zhang LH, Zhang YC, Wang YJ, *et al.* Efficacy observation on Governor Vessel-regulating and brain-unblocking acupuncture for post-stroke depression. J Acup Tuina Sci, 2016, 14(3): 175-180

[77] Mao ZN, He TY, Mao LY. Clinic study of the treatment of post-stroke difficulty of swallow with "target acupuncture" method of Prof. He Tian-You. TCM annual conference of Gansu province, China, 2015

[78] Li MY, Zu W, Sun XW. Clinic observation of the treatment of post-stroke insomnia with Tong Luo An Shen method of acupuncture. Acup Clinic J. 2016; 32(4):31-33

[79] Yu C, Shen B, Xu SW, Xu YP. Efficacy observation of Yi Shen Tong Qiao acupuncture in the treatment of post-stroke difficulty of swallow and life quality. Modern distance education of Chinese Medicine. 2016; 14(10): 46-48

[80] Hao LX, Zhang JY, Jia YJ. Clinic experience of Li Ji Chun in the treatment of stroke. World J integrated traditional Chinese and Western Medicine. 2016; 11(6):778-780

[81] Ding BY, Duan JY, Zhou YL, Cao XW. Treatment of post-stroke upper limb paralysis with Chou Qian method of Acupuncture. World J Acup-Moxi. 2016. 26(2):31-36

[82] Meng FZ, Li P. Example in the clinic treatment with "Tong Du Tiao Shen' style of acupuncture by Prof. Li Ping.
http://www.wfas.org.cn/lunwen/wfas20/201108/2871.html

[83] Gao HM, Fu Y. Brief theoretical discussion for the "Shallow stimulation with needle on skin layer" proposed by Professor Fu Yu. TCM clinical Res. 2016;8(19):57-59

[84] Huang DT, Pang SH, Zhou CH, Lu YY, Jiang RZ, Liao LL, Wu W, Yu TZ. Influence and Evaluation on Effects of Rehabilitation in 50 cases of Spastic Hemiplegia of Stroke Treated by Skin Surface Acupuncture with Medicated Thread Moxibustion. Acup Clin J. 2012; 28(10):18-20

[85] Yan MX, Yu Y. Curative Effects of Combining Cutaneous Needling with Five - elements Music on 63 Depressive Patients with Heart -spleen Deficiency. Acup Clinic J. 2016;32(1):11-14

[86] Liu CC, Fu Y. The experience in the treatment of allergic nasitis by Professor Fu Yu with shallow stimulation on skin with acupuncture. Shanxi TCM. 2016;32(9): 14-15

[87] Chen DC. Overall introduction of "Dong Jin Acupuncture" and targets of treatment. Chinese Acup & Moxi. 2016; 36(9):941-944

[88] Guan WQ, Zhen RN, Cui SM, Fan JY. Introduction of the "Nu Yun Zhi Zhen" acupuncture method by Professor Lu Mei in the treatment of chronic elbow pain syndrome. China J Chinese Med. 2013; 4:514-515

[89] Zhang TS, Nie PR, Guan F, Wen H. Brief discussion about the "Yi Tong Zhu Ten" acupuncture technique introduced by Professor Wen Hong. China Naturopathy. 2014. 22(1): 8-9

[90] Baidu Baike website. Introduction of Around Acupuncture.
http://baike.baidu.com/view/3508557.htm

[91] Dong's Acupuncture main website. http://www.tungs.net.cn/zh-tw/

[92] Wu Yong-Xiang. Introduction and discussion questions about Dong's extraordinary acupuncture points and traditional Chinese acupuncture by Dr. Yang Wei Jie. http://www.360doc.com/content/11/0903/18/7644441_145527152.shtml

[93] Peterjo. Christ-Western medicine-Chinese medicine – Distance Luo Medicine. http://blog.xuite.net/peterjo/diary/69247612-%E5%9F%BA%E7%9D%A3%E4%B8%AD%E8%A5%BF%E9%86%AB%E5%AD%B8-%E9%81%A0%E7%B5%A1%E9%86%AB%E5%AD%B8

[94] Zhou XG. Difference between the Luo points in the Distance-Luo acupuncture and traditional Chinese Luo points. http://blog.xuite.net/hannah716/twblog/158411212-%E9%81%A0%E7%B5%A1%E7%99%82%E6%B3%95%E7%B5%A1%E7%A9%B4%E5%92%8C%E5%82%B3%E7%B5%B1%E4%B8%AD%E9%86%AB%E7%B5%A1%E7%A9%B4%E6%87%89%E7%94%A8%E7%9A%84%E5%B7%AE%E5%88%A5

[95] Pain treatment center, Tri Service General Hospital. Notice for use of the Distance-luo acupressure treatment. http://wwwu.tsgh.ndmctsgh.edu.tw/ane/pain/enrac.html

[96] Lin FX. Brief introduction of Distance-lou acupressure therapy.http://windfix.pixnet.net/blog/post/316721364-%E6%9F%AF%E6%B0%8F%E9%81%A0%E7%B5%A1%E7%99%82%E6%B3%95%E7%B0%A1%E4%BB%8B

[97] Guo M, Yang SJ, Chen HD. Therapeutic Observation of Distant Collateral Needling for Cervical Spondylotic Radiculopath. Shanghai J Acup & Moxi. 2016; 35(9):1109-1111

[98] Xuite. Christ-Western medicine-Chinese medicine – Distance Luo Medicine. http://blog.xuite.net/peterjo/diary/69247612-%E5%9F%BA%E7%9D%A3%E4%B8%AD%E8%A5%BF%E9%86%AB%E5%AD%B8-%E9%81%A0%E7%B5%A1%E9%86%AB%E5%AD%B8

[99] Wu SQ. Introduction of the experience in use of "One-needle acupuncture therapy" introduced by Han Wen Zhi. World Chinese Med. 2008; 3: 153-155 Supplement.

[100] Wu SQ. Introduction of the "Twelve birth-animal-symbol acupuncture therapy" introduced by Han Wen Zhi. World Chinese Med. 2008; 3: 58 Supplement.

[101] Wu SQ. Summary of the experience in the treatment of hypertension with the acupuncture style introduced by Dr. Han Wen-Zhi. http://www.hkjtcm.org/journals/2011%E5%B9%B4%E7%AC%AC%E5%85%AD%E5%8D%B7%E7%AC%AC%E4%B8%80%E6%9C%9F/18.%20%E5%8F%B0%E7%81%A3%E9%9F%93%E6%96%87%E6%B2%BB%E9%87%9D%E6%B3%95%E6%B2%BB%E7%99%82%E9%AB%98%E8%A1%80%E5%A3%93%E7%97%85%E7%9A%84%E7%B6%93%E9%A9%97%E5%BD%99%E7%B2%B9.pdf

[102] Zhang XS. Practical Wrist-Ankle Acupuncture. People's Medical Publishing House. 2003

[103] Wrist-ankle. Acupuncturehttp://www.baike.com/ wiki/%E8%85%95%E8%B8%9D%E9%92%88%E6%B3%95

[104] Wang GQ. Technique handbook for Chinese medicine therapies. World Federation of acupuncture and Moxibustion Societies. http://mp.weixin.qq.com/s?__biz=MzA3MTMxNjMwOA==&mid=2694210277&idx=8 &sn=73001420a2cea562b5174e37448338d2&scene=0#wechat_redirect

[105] White A. Western medical acupuncture: a definition. Acup Med. 2009 Mar;27(1):33-5. doi: 10.1136/aim.2008.000372.

[106] Website for Chinese medicine development. Auricular Acupuncture. http://www.wfas.org.cn/tcmtools/therapy/820.html

[107] Ear Acupuncture Chart. http://lwk.yes1798.com/lwk/search/view.asp?RecordNo=50943&NAME=%C2%A6%C3%95%C2%A5%C3%9E%C2%B9%C3%8F

[108] Zhao CH, Fan GQ, Zhao Y. Comparison and development of different scalp needling schools. Chinese Acup & Moxi. 2016: 36(6):663-667

[109] Huaxia Jingwei website. Acupuncture- Scalp Acupuncture. http://big5.huaxia.com/hxjk/zhyx/zjtn/2009/06/1453618.html

[110] Baidu Baike. Scalp Acupuncture Therapy. http://baike.baidu.com/view/832430.htm

[111] Qiu YF. Acupuncture treatment for stroke: Scalp Acupuncture. http://blog.xuite.net/strokeonline/info/154742430-%E9%87%9D%E7%81%B8%E6%B2%BB%E7%99%82%E4%B8%AD%E9%A2%A8+-+%E9%A0%AD%E9%87%9D%E7%AF%87

[112] Zhu MQ. China Folk Chinese medicine development association. Introduction of Dr. Zhu Mingqing. http://www.guanliao.net/terminfo.asp?id=16

[113] Huaxia Chinese Medicine Glory website. Traditional Chinese Medicine: Acupuncture. http://www.uuchatroom.com/zhenjiu/3363223.html

[114] Ye MZ, Tang HX. Dr. Tang Yan-Tin and his "Tang's Scalp Acupuncture Therapy". J TCM Literature. 2010;28(2):50-54

[115] Wenku website. New acupuncture points on Ling Xue-Jian style of Scalp acupuncture. http://wenku.todgo.com/nonglinmuyu/59949791ede54.html

[116] Yu CD, Wu BH, Chen Y, Liu K, Chen XJ, Zhang GF. Application anatomy of acupuncture on skull suture for treatment of cerebrovascular diseases. Chinese Acup & Moxi. 2002;22(3):177-179 .

[117] Shouxi Medicine Website. The clinical experience of professor Jin Rui. http://journal.9med.net/html/qikan/lcyx/zhxdlcyxzz/2005131/zyzy/20080901061327145_66342.html

[118] China national Chinese medicine library. New Scalp Acupuncture of Toshikatsu Yamamoto. http://lib.cintcm.ac.cn:8089/opac/book/314985

[119] Baidu Baike. Facial Acupuncture. http://baike.baidu.com/view/6935328.htm

[120] Huang YL. Introduction of new facial acupuncture. http://www.cdutcm.com/post/1532.html

[121] Fu WB. Eye acupuncture therapy and its clinical application. http://www.hnzjxh.com/onews.asp?id=26

[122] Wu Dao Xiu Xing. Eye acupuncture: diagnosis from eyes introduced by professor Peng Jing-Shan. http://www.360doc.com/content/14/0227/17/9774604_356208274.shtml

[123] Beike.com. Eye Acupuncture Therapy. http://www.baike.com/wiki/%E7%9C%BC%E9%92%88%E7%96%97%E6%B3%95

[124] Five-Taste Master. Eye Acupuncture. http://www.360doc.com/content/09/0817/21/203041_4999945.shtml

[125] Baike.com. Nose Acupuncture. http://www.baike.com/wiki/%E9%BC%BB%E9%92%88%E7%96%97%E6%B3%95

[126] Tang Han Chinese Medicine website. Acupuncture points in nose acupuncture system. http://book.th55.cn/a/200903/6456.html

[127] Baike.com. Tongue Acupuncture. http://www.baike.com/wiki/%E8%88%8C%E9%92%88%E7%96%97%E6%B3%95

[128] Liu HX. Introduction of mouth acupuncture system. http://blog.sina.com.cn/u/1559311971

[129] Jialove333. Mouth Acupuncture. http://www.documentsky.com/752668353/

[130] Baike.com. Introduction of Ren-zhong Acupuncture.
http://www.baike.com/wiki/%E4%BA%BA%E4%B8%AD%E9%92%88%E7%96%97%E6%B3%95

[131] Acupuncture China website. Application of Modern Acupuncture and Moxibustion: Feet Acupuncture. http://www.acucn.com/college/technique/200704/3032.html

[132] Medical Encyclopedia website. Introduction of Feet Acupuncture therapy.
http://www.wiki8.com/zuzhenliaofa_119798/

[133] Xue B. Cited from Dou-Ding website. Hand diagram and Feet diagram – creation by Dr. Fang (2). http://www.360doc.com/content/17/0112/23/20699624_622105952.shtml

[134] Tang Han Chinese Medicine website. Feet Diagram Acupuncture.
http://book.th55.cn/a/200902/4194.html

[135] Pharmaceutical drug development center of Zhong Shan University. Acupuncture points on back of hands, for Hand acupuncture system.
http://www.ddcd120.com/content/?777.html

[136] Wuji 8 website. Reactive point chart for Hand acupuncture system.
http://www.wuji8.com/meta/429084912.html

[137] 51yam.com. Introduction of the Yin-Yang nine acupuncture by Yu Hao.
http://www.51yam.com/thread-256316-1-1.html

[138] Ping Kang Tang Massage. The Yin-Yang nine acupuncture system by Dr. Yu in Ren-zhi-tang clinic center.
http://www.360doc.com/content/16/0628/12/5620517_571355557.shtml

[139] Ge QF. Taiji Six He Acupuncture. http://baike.baidu.com/view/2509798.htm

[140] Fu Xin TCM website. My understanding about the Eight words therapy.
http://www.helpweixin.com/html/229496.html

[141] H Zhu Q website cited. Ma Chun-Hui. Open the mysterious veil of Small Six-He acupuncture . http://www.360doc.com/content/14/1211/15/11285146_432153121.shtml

[142] Easy Life website. Palm Eight Diagram – watch your health.
http://e1689.blogspot.ca/2012/07/blog-post.html

[143] Hong Yi Tang. Hong Yi Continuous introduction: Nan Hai-Jin: Yijing explanation.
http://www.hyt2000.com/resource01.php?pid=44&PHPSESSID=c7b5e5bc18baaef601efbe35d7fe5f4e

[144] Ren Zhe Ai Ren. Mysterious Taiji Six-He Acupuncture.
http://www.360doc.com/content/11/0218/19/619786_94138035.shtml

[145] Chen F. Abdominal Acupuncture system.
http://www.360doc.com/content/10/0716/21/474297_39512983.shtml

[146] xyf4345. Abdominal Acupuncture: Valuable material in Acupuncture study.
http://www.360doc.com/content/16/0816/23/29553696_583739407.shtml

[147] Xing Ji. Book information: Comments on the Clinic case report for abdominal acupuncture. http://www.360doc.com/content/15/0224/15/11605768_450478906.shtml

[148] Xu PK. Abdominal Acupuncture (Summary of academic experience of Dr. Sun Shen-Tian). Heilongjian University TCM. Ph. D. Thesis, April, 2006.

[149] Sun YZ, Yu T. Clinical Research on the First Area of Sun's Abdominal Acupuncture Treatment for Insomnia. JCAM. 2014;30(12):42-44

[150] Shen GB, Wang J, Shi S. Clinic observation on the treatment of insomnia with Sun's Abdominal acupuncture and Four-gate points. World Latest Medicine Information. 2014; 14(34):277

[151] Da Hai Chinese Medicine. Introduction of the first developer of Navel acupuncture, the Yi medicine master- Prof. Qi Yong.
http://blog.sina.com.cn/s/blog_60a4a9bb0100e30a.html

[152] Dong ZH, Qi Y. Navel Acupuncture. Chinese Acup & Moxi. 2002; 22(8): 570-571

[153] Jun Lin Tian Xia 177 Website. Time Medicine, Six Jing Diagnosis and Navel Acupuncture. http://www.360doc.com/content/16/0412/02/14001169_549872594.shtml

[154] He JJ. The relationship between the Chinese medicine and Eight Diagram.
http://www.hkama.hk/journal/journal0901/content06/c6_01.htm

[155] Winnie. Introduction of earth branch in Time Medicine.
http://baike.haoyun666.com/index.php?doc-view-629.htm

[156] Good relationship physio-therapy. Talk about Navel Acupuncture by Navel Acupuncture expert. http://www.shanyuankang.com/html/zwll/zjcx/2707.html

[157] Mountain Water Master. The positive reactive organ reflecting points in 《Biological Holographic therapy》. http://blog.sina.com.cn/s/blog_5ff306380102uwd8.html

[158] Okboy website. Holographic acupuncture point chart on second metacarpale and its secrete in treatment. http://www.360doc.com/content/09/0326/17/73907_2926067.shtml

[159] Med66.com. The Holographic acupuncture point chart in fifth metacarpale. http://www.med66.com/new/42a206a2010/2010111zhangf165224.shtml

[160] Ma Wang website: "Nine-palace Acupuncture therapy. http://blog.sina.com.cn/s/blog_89da3dfe0101b4aj.html

[161] Wang XL. Learning from Feng Han Ning about Nine-palace Acupuncture. http://www.hztjt.com/MEMBER/Views/1387

[162] Zhao M, Wang XY. Nine-palace Acupuncture treatment of 100 cases of prolapse of lumbar intervertebral disc. Yunnan J TCM and Materia Medica. 2012;33(5):84

[163] Guan ZH. Clinic application of hot needle in spine Nine-palace acupuncture. http://zhongyibaodian.com/yianxinde/76005.html

[164] Chen GL. Treatment of 526 cases of prolapse of lumbar intervertebral disc with spine Nine-palace acupuncture plus cupping therapy. Chinese Folk Therapy. 2008;8:24

[165] Yin XC. Nine acupuncture needles and twelve methods. http://www.jzsef.com/view.php?ID=227

[166] Yin XC. Treatment of prolapse of lumbar intervertebral disc with Nine acupuncture needles and twelve methods. http://www.huaxiamingyi.com/mylt/20130407/105437.aspx

[167] Zhang WB, Huo ZJ. Muscle starting-end point therapy – Releasing point therapy. People 's Health Publishing House, 2005

[168] Xian Zai Ju Shi website: Releasing point – Muscle starting-end point therapy and its clinical application. http://blog.sina.com.cn/s/blog_6383a68a0102e50g.html

[169] Shen Wei-Yi website. Understanding muscle trigger point- knowing more introduction.. http://weibo.com/ttarticle/p/show?id=2309404025714667093284

[170] Qi F. The "Trigger point" of muscle-tendon pain syndrome. http://blog.sina.com.cn/s/blog_5433aa7b0100m1wx.html

[171] Liu NY, Ren TP, Xiang Y. Immediate analgesic effects of tendon acupuncture on soft tissue injury. Chinese Acup & Moxi. 2015; 35(9): 927-929

[172] Xing Lin Ya Shi website. No Pain Acupuncture. http://www.360doc.com/content/11/0601/21/840524_121045242.shtml

[173] Itoh K, Kitakoji H. Acupuncture for chronic pain in Japan: a review. Evid Based Complement Alternat Med. 2007 Dec;4(4):431-8

[174] Xun Tian Yuan cited from Sina Blog: New recognition and new application of the nature of acupuncture points and its relationship with inner organs.http://www.360doc.com/content/14/1223/13/7470776_435154741.shtml

[175] Fei L, Ding GH, Shen XY, Gu QB, Chen EY. Exploration of the material basis and functional characteristics of meridians. Bulletin of advanced technology research. 2011;5(3):6-8

[176] Zhang LQ. The nature of meridian is the brain information controlling system of body. World Health Digest. 2012;6:237-239

[177] Zhen X. The characteristics and current situations of major styles of acupuncture in US. Beijing Univ. TCM. Ph. D. Thesis. 2012